SURVIVING ADVERSITY

living with Parkinson's disease

Book and Cover Design by: MacMillan Marketing Group Inc.

www.SurvivingAdversity.com

Printed and bound in Canada, First Printing March 2007

Library and Archives Canada Cataloguing in Publication

Carley, Gord, 1962-

    Surviving adversity : living with Parkinson's disease / Gord Carley.

Includes index.
ISBN 978-0-9734162-1-3

    1. Parkinson's disease - Patients - Biography.
    I.Title. II. Title: Living with Parkinson's disease.

RC382.C382 2007 362.196'83300922 C2007-900734-1

Please note: Surviving Adversity—living with Parkinson's disease does not advocate, endorse or promote any drug therapy, course of treatment, surgical procedure or specific company or institution. It is strongly recommended that care and treatment decisions related to Parkinson's disease and any other medical condition be made in consultation with a patient's physician or other qualified medical professionals.

OVERVIEW—Parkinson's disease

What is Parkinson's disease?
Parkinson's disease is a brain disorder. It occurs when certain nerve cells (neurons) in a part of the brain called the *substantia nigra* die or become impaired. Normally, these cells produce a vital chemical known as dopamine, which allows smooth, coordinated function of the body's muscles and movement. When approximately 80% of the dopamine-producing cells are damaged, the symptoms of Parkinson's disease appear.

Symptoms of Parkinson's disease:
Symptoms vary from person to person. Classic signs of the disease are tremors, slowness of movement, rigidity, and problems with balance. Depression is also common. Other signs include a stiff facial expression, muffled speech, small handwriting and difficulty walking.

Who gets Parkinson's disease?
In North America it is estimated that 1.5 million people have Parkinson's disease. It affects 1 of every 100 people over the age of 60. Men are slightly more prone than females to get Parkinson's disease. On average, it usually develops after the age of 60 although approximately 15% of patients have been diagnosed before the age of 50.

Cause of Parkinson's disease:
The exact cause(s) of Parkinson's disease is not known. It is believed that environmental and genetic factors play a role but currently there are no definitive statistics on the possible causes.

Cure for Parkinson's disease:
Research is currently being conducted throughout the world, analyzing the disease from many angles. At this point, there is no cure for Parkinson's disease.

CONTENTS

CONTENTS

CONTENTS

CONTENTS

ACKNOWLEDGEMENTS

Welcome to *Surviving Adversity—living with Parkinson's disease.* I hope that this book will motivate and encourage others, especially those who are going through a difficult time—as well as increase awareness of Parkinson's disease.

I would like to thank everyone whose profile appears in this book for sharing their stories and contributing thoughts, ideas and anecdotes—both verbally and in written form.

The following people have all taken time to help me—their support is much appreciated:

Brooke Ballantyne, Kim Barnett, Bill Bell, Paul Blom, Diane Breslow, Jim Canto, Carey Christensen, Vicki Conte, Grant Cranston, Adolfo Diaz, Rena Dohm, Peter Dunlap-Shohl, Melany Ethridge, Ruth Hagestuen, Brenda Harris, Carole Hartzman, Bill Heinmiller, Gordon & Judy Hiebert, Jan Humphreys, Ron James, John Kraft, Charlene Lustig, Christine MacGregor, Sarah Magee, Diane McQuiston, Sharon Metz, Alan Muir, Nick Peterson, Sheri Rapp, Donna Redman, Tanya Riemann, Jo Rosen, Barbara Snelgrove, Mary Ann Sprinkle, Ann Staton, Greg and Kathy Stiffler, Carolyn Stinson, Nicole Teed, Tim Thaler, Paula Tomlin, David Von Hofen, Jane Widdecombe, Jim Williams, Marjie Zacks and Jean Zwolinski.

Many organizations have been very helpful to me—two especially: The National Parkinson Foundation (NPF) and the Parkinson Society Canada (PSC). Their assistance has been invaluable.

A very special thanks goes to my brother Dave for his help in editing. It's a nice windfall to have a brother who is a playwright and also has over 30 years of editing experience in newspapers and radio drama. Thank you also to Jenn Harris and Katherine Hanz—both of whom have diligently read through stories and patiently corrected my excessive use of some forms of punctuation.

Without the advice, understanding and support of my wife Andra, this book would not have been completed. My children, Meg and Walter, have helped in their own way by always keeping me smiling and entertained.

From a broader perspective, I also want to recognize the caregivers, support organizations, medical professionals, and researchers who are all working to make the lives of those afflicted more comfortable. Finally, I salute the 1.5 million courageous people in North America—and the millions more throughout the world—who battle Parkinson's disease on a daily basis.

INTRODUCTION

One of the most inspiring individuals I know—and the one who has had the greatest influence on me is my mother, Margaret. She was diagnosed with Parkinson's disease in 2002, and she is the catalyst for my writing this book.

My mother grew up in Peterborough, Ontario. She attended McGill University in Montreal and, after graduating, moved to Toronto. There she worked in the Department of Preventive Medicine at the University of Toronto for six years and, during that time, earned a Master's degree in Microbiology. My mother and father were married in 1949 and, after Dad graduated from law school, they moved back to Peterborough. Dad entered his father's law firm and Mom stayed home full-time, raising four children.

My father died in 1983, when I was 20 years old. I had been very close to him and, up to that point, my mother had always been—well, a mother. She looked after me, disciplined me, and also seemed to do one thousand things all at once. After my dad died, the relationship between my mother and me expanded. She has continued to play the mother role to perfection, but she has also become my most trusted friend—I can talk to her about anything. From time to time, she has heard me vent about something and then offered advice that proved to be wiser than the action that I wanted to pursue. She is lots of fun but also a bit of a worrier—I still have letters on the benefits of eating balanced meals that she sent to me during the time when I was eating pizza every other night and consuming about four bowls of cereal a day.

A few years ago, I noticed that her multitasking skills were slipping a bit. It took her longer to get ready for things. Her walk became stiff and she seemed to tire more frequently. At the age of 78, she determined the reason—self-diagnosing that she had Parkinson's disease after researching it on the Internet. Her family doctor and a neurosurgeon confirmed her diagnosis. Since then, my mother has slowed down somewhat and she is not physically as strong as she once was. However, she has not let that stand in the way of living her life. She enjoys her local support group as well as a weekly Parkinson's exercise class and, with the help of her medications, she continues to live independently.

I dedicate this book to my mother, Margaret Carley.

CHAPTER ONE

DAVIS PHINNEY

"Every victory counts!"

Davis Phinney was diagnosed with Parkinson's disease in 2000. He is 47 years old.

When I was 15 years old, I was a little lost and unsure of who I was or what I wanted to do, and I was somewhat disenchanted with many things. A bicycle race came to town, and so I went to the local park and stood at the fence that lined the course. I watched these guys go around and around—it was like magic. There was so much speed, energy, fluidity, color and even drama in the couple of hours that I watched these riders flying by me. Seeing that race was the right thing to inspire me at the right time. I was extremely pumped and I rode my junky ten-speed bike home and told myself that I was going to be a bike racer. The course of my life was irrevocably changed at that point and I committed myself to becoming a professional cyclist.

Racing at the highest levels of the sport—riding in the Tour de France and throughout Europe in particular—led to me facing my share of adversity in the competitive realm. As a rider, you are faced with challenges from the weather, the competition, the terrain, the distance of the race, or all of these. On flat ground, I would be going at 25 miles per hour, and downhill I might reach speeds of 60 miles per hour. Fatigue and self-doubt constantly have to be overcome. Some races can become quite an ordeal. For example, two and half weeks into a race like the Tour de France, a typical day starts with you being dead tired and facing a ride of over two hundred kilometers with four major climbs. In addition, you have got to get to the finish line in a time that is in close proximity to the winner or you are eliminated, which is called 'making the time limit'. But it is in persevering and making it through those hard days in the Tour that you define your capabilities. My cycling experience gave me the confidence that I could handle any challenge I would face in the future. Little did I know what was waiting for me.

Towards the end of my cycling career, I started to have troubles with my left leg and I frequently had to stretch it to keep it from cramping. I figured it had to be some physiological issue from training, so I spent a lot of time on the massage table. After retiring from competitive cycling, I took on many jobs and I became extremely fatigued. Basically, I ground myself down. The problems with my leg were increasing—my foot started to cramp up when I was running, and I started tripping and dragging my leg. This went on for years. Over time, the muscle cramping moved up to my left forearm and hand. I started to get a noticeable tremor ten years after I had the first symptoms. I had minor tremors before that time but assumed that they were because I was too tired. But then one day, while I was holding a microphone trying to do a television interview, my tremors became uncontrollable—I couldn't ignore the problem any longer. I knew I had to determine what was causing these symptoms.

It took a long time to diagnose me because the neurologists in town did not think of me as a candidate for Parkinson's. It wore me out talking to doctors, getting MRIs and going for seemingly every test known to man. I started to search online and found a Parkinson's young-onset website and it had a checklist. Eight out of ten symptoms noted on that checklist fit me, which was my first inkling that I might have Parkinson's disease. Finally a friend of mine, Andy Pruitt, who runs the Boulder Center for Sports Medicine, sent me to a venerable old-school neurologist who put me through the paces before giving me the correct diagnosis and telling me that I had Parkinson's.

Upon hearing the diagnosis, my wife and I came back to Boulder. I did three shots of tequila and I thought, "Okay, here is a life changing experience." I was fairly dejected at first but also a little relieved to know what I had, even though I did not know much about the disease. I was pretty well-known in the community, so there had been a lot of speculation about my condition. I did a news conference where I stated that I had Parkinson's disease. At that point my symptoms were fairly minimal, so everyone was saying, "You look fine" or "You look great" and even, "I think I had a little problem like that, too." When I heard those things, I thought to myself, "If you think you are helping me by saying that, you are not doing a good job."

After I went public, various people in the Parkinson's community descended on me to get me to jump in and help the cause, but I was not yet ready for that, as I did not understand the disease or how my future would be affected by living with it. Also, my father, whose fifteen-year battle with cancer had been a great inspiration to me and many others, had come out of remission and his health declined rapidly on the heels of my diagnosis. For much of the next year I was involved in taking care of him until his death in the fall of 2001. After he passed away, I started to muse about how to turn my situation into an opportunity. My wife and I had always dreamed of taking the kids to live abroad, so we quickly decided to move to Italy. We lived there for three years and it was a wonderful respite. We found a small town where I could be anonymous, a place where I was simply the shaky American down the street. Ultimately, this time away led me to accept the disease and helped me to decide how I could best make a contribution to the cause—and that in turn led to us starting our own foundation.

Currently, I am focused on doing everything I can do to improve my overall health, much in the way I once went about attaining my athletic goals. In this way, I truly believe I am minimizing my symptoms and slowing my rate of decline. I'm pursuing a combination of both alternative and mainstream methodologies. For example, after five years of being Sinemet-free, I started to take the drug, but I also see an acupuncturist. As well, I cook up Chinese herbs each day—a Western/Eastern medicinal blend which I find really helps.

In the past, my lifestyle combined with Parkinson's disease dragged my whole energy level so far down that I felt I was behind ten years worth of sleep. Slowly, I have brought myself back to a more energized place. I drink a super nutrient green drink each morning, and I do a whole host of core body strengthening, stretching, and balancing exercises almost every day. I also believe that sweating is a key component in detoxifying the body and promoting healthy cell turnover, and have installed an infrared sauna in our house, which I use regularly. I ride bikes, ski and take frequent hikes—all helpful and healthy activities. Granted, I can no longer exercise anywhere near the levels I once did but I am a huge proponent of the benefits that exercise provides. All of these things can be easy to forego but that's where my athletic background comes in handy, as I've got an ingrained discipline to follow the process consistently to achieve the desired result.

I am very much into positive self-motivation. It is so easy to become negative when you have this disease—it is easy to be negative anytime—but in living with Parkinson's you get so frustrated because simple things can be a big challenge. But the way I look at it is, if I can get my shirt buttoned then I have just scored a victory. When I was competitively racing, regardless of what went right or what went wrong throughout the race, as long as I could get across the finish line first and throw my arms up in the air, that was an immediate gratification and a payoff for all the effort. I still focus on victories and the payoff, only now the victories are of a different sort. Each little moment that you can denote as something positive in your day must be acknowledged as a victory. For example, when my daughter runs up and gives me a big hug—that is an absolute victory. Every victory counts!

My advice is to become as knowledgeable as you can about Parkinson's but not to become obsessed about when a cure or medical wonder is going to happen. The medical wonder that you can affect is in your daily approach to managing your disease and that includes both physical and mental aspects. Focus on the positive, acknowledge your victories and make every day a good day.

I think what happens quite frequently when you have a disabling disease is that you stop being able to see the forest because the tree is right in your face all the time. You don't step back and approach things differently because you are so close to that dumb tree. All you see are the shadows of the disease and its effects on you. That type of tunnel vision ends up bringing you down and that accelerates your decline —plus you drive away everyone who cares about you.

One of the huge challenges with this disease is getting out into public. It is very enticing to hide in the closet because you don't want to be with people and you don't want others to judge you. However, the primary source of energy in life is interacting with people and getting energy from them. I feel that if you can become a positive person despite your own issues or disabilities then you will attract positive energy. If I go out and I'm in a bad mood I will not receive good energy in return. But when I go out and I am smiling and engaged with people, regardless of whether I am shaky or not, then I always come home feeling good and tanked up with energy.

Get the knowledge you need so that you can become as healthy as possible. That will allow you to regain some of your function, which will help you to regain some of your confidence, which in turn will help you get out in public and also enjoy your life.

Believe in yourself and don't give up. Take ownership of your obligations as a person with Parkinson's disease and do everything you can to improve your life right now. Do not wait and hold out hope that someone else will fix your problem. There is a lot we can do for ourselves.

Between the late 1970s and 1993, Davis Phinney won 328 races–more than any other U.S. cyclist. He also won a Bronze Medal in the 1984 Olympics. Davis Phinney, Lance Armstrong and Greg LeMond are the only Americans to win multiple stages of the Tour de France, bicycle racing's premiere event.

After retiring, Davis Phinney was a sportscaster for ABC, CBS, NBC and OLN. He now devotes his time to The Davis Phinney Foundation (DPF). The objective of the DPF is "To fund research that validates and develops cure-like treatment options to slow or even halt the progression of Parkinson's disease and extend a patient's quality of life. Ultimately, we believe our collective scientific contribution will help accelerate the progress towards finding a cure to this debilitating disease."

CHAPTER TWO

PAT HULL

"I'm sorry, I keep getting so distracted by all of your arms and legs that I forget to watch you walk."

Pat Hull was diagnosed with Parkinson's disease in April 2001. She is 67 years old.

My children think of me as 'somewhat eccentric' but I prefer the phrase 'free thinker'. I completed high school and got married at age 18, was divorced at 30, remarried at 31, and divorced again at age 59. I am the mother of four children, grandmother of sixteen and great-grandmother of five. My two eldest children are from my first marriage and they are old enough to be the two youngest children's parents.

My youngest daughter contracted Acute Lymphocytic Leukemia *(ALL)* in 1982. She was three years old at the time. I quit work to care for her while she endured four years of chemotherapy and subsequent therapy for years after that. She turned out to be a rare ALL patient—she is still alive today. Having lived through that situation helped to give me perspective in my current battle with Parkinson's.

In 2001, I was living in Phoenix. I put my name on match.com (*an online dating service*) and a number of gentlemen called me for dates. One man took me to a Chinese restaurant. It was a cold evening and it was chilly in the restaurant, too. I was having a terrible time eating my soup—I was shaking and spilling quite a bit. I attributed it to the frigid temperature of the restaurant. My date was watching me and he pointedly commented, "I could never take you to a business dinner—you can't even manage soup." He left rather abruptly once our meal was finished.

I returned to my home after the date and I soon realized that something else might be the cause of my shaking hand, because it was still happening in the warmth of my house. I went to my primary care physician and said, "I'm having this problem with my hand—it keeps shaking." She referred me to a neurologist who, after thoroughly examining me, said, "I think you have Parkinson's, but the best way we can tell is if the medication I prescribe helps to stop your shaking." I took the Parkinson's medicine and it worked. I was diagnosed in April 2001, just a few weeks after my date at the Chinese restaurant.

The doctor gave me a booklet about Parkinson's and I spent two days doing some intense introspection. I wasn't a very happy camper during that time, but I'm not a person who stays down for long. I soon decided, "I have got it and I'll deal with it. Time to get back to my normal life."

Then an amazing thing happened. In January 2006, Stanley, a 71-year-old man that I had met the previous June through an ad in a seniors' publication, declared his love for me.

We agreed upon a 'lifelong engagement/arrangement', and he moved in with me. I was very pleasantly surprised that anyone would commit to a long-term relationship with me, considering my health conditions.

Stanley and I have almost nothing in common except ill health, aging, and an appreciation of Chinese take-out food. This has allowed us to introduce each other to a fascinating array of 'new' things. Jewish and Brooklyn-born, Stanley has taken me to Jewish restaurants for chopped liver and lox, while I have exposed him to Southwestern U.S. foods. He tolerates my love of Native American art and the fact that it fills our house. He collects baseball cards and I am learning to appreciate the game, too. Life is good. I have someone to cook for, care for, to be with, laugh with and lie close to in bed. I feel needed and useful again.

Stanley is like a teenager in a car—there is only one speed, and that's 'go'. He is like a whirling dervish, because he never stops—he just goes from one thing to another. Stanley has more health issues than I do, but he does not let them affect how he lives life. He is very enthusiastic about everything he tackles and his enthusiasm is contagious. I just follow him around—the exercise involved in just doing that is wonderful.

One time, around Halloween, I had an appointment with a neurologist, so Stanley and I decided to dress up and go to the office in our costumes. The office staff and the nurses went wild when they saw us and they all laughed hysterically. Stanley was outfitted in a Superman costume, complete with a red cape and a 16-inch-tall Marge Simpson wig on his head. I was a six-legged bumblebee with white gauzy wings and glittery green antennae. When I finally got in to see the doctor, he made me walk up and down the hall three times. The doctor apologized, saying, "I'm sorry, I keep getting so distracted by all of your arms and legs that I forget to watch you walk."

We love animals and birds. Stanley has a couple of parakeets, three finches, and a dozen cockatiels. We raised eight chickens, incubating them in the bathtub with a light hanging off the shower to keep them warm. Now they are grown up and laying eggs like crazy. My 'pet' is a wolf hybrid that is part Lobo wolf and part Malamute. He weighs 115 pounds and he is very dear to me. He looks just like a calendar picture of a wolf. He doesn't bark, but he makes some sounds that come close to barking. However, whenever a fire engine goes by with its siren blaring, it is like 'call of the wild'—he tilts his head back and howls.

Donna Redman is a professor from Arizona State University and also a volunteer who has done a lot to help Parkinson's patients in our area. She runs an annual, sixteen-week program that takes place on Saturdays. One time, she asked us to write down anything in our life that we would like to do or learn, and she said that she would try to make it happen. I had always wished that I had learned the art of tatting (*an ancient lace-making technique*) from my mother, so I listed that. About halfway through the next week's meeting, Donna gave me a VCR tape. It turns out that she had stayed up quite late one night in order to tape a PBS broadcast on tatting. She has been a huge inspiration to me.

There is always a way to get something done. I wanted to paint a mural of Monument Valley on the bathroom wall—however, I don't have very good balance. I figured that there must be a way to do it. The solution that I found was a really neat ladder—it has wide steps and a big loop at the top, so that I can climb up and paint the tops of the walls without the risk of falling off the ladder. I can paint much better in the morning when I'm fresh—by the afternoon, I tend to have a little down time and that makes for wavy lines. The mural is almost done and I'm very pleased with the result.

I'm retired, and the nice thing about being retired is that you can be impulsive. If you wake up in the morning and you want to go somewhere, you can. If you want to sleep in, you can. I've decided that I am not making too many long-term plans but that is not just because I have Parkinson's. I have made long-term plans in my life before and I have often found them cut short by other events. For example, I had planned a career in real estate which did not end up happening because of my daughter's leukemia. I had planned to have a much more posh retirement with perhaps some foreign travel, but that failed to materialize because of my divorce. In my opinion, there is no such thing as long-term security. Change brings growth, so who really needs security? I live much more in the moment now than I used to.

I sing all the time, especially in the car. I like to sing a lot of songs from American musicals and also songs that I learned during my many years as a Girl Scout volunteer. You can't be unhappy when you are singing, can you?

I think it is very important to educate yourself about your medications. Don't be afraid to say "No" or even to switch doctors if you are uncomfortable with a new treatment or medication that is being prescribed by your doctor or neurologist. It is your body—not theirs.

Worry is a waste of time and energy. You just have to look to the future and deal with it. When something happens to you that isn't pleasant, you can choose to continue on, stand up and do things and have a good time, or you can quit and wilt. It is definitely your choice. It's what we choose to do with our time here that's important. We can waste our energy with self-pity, addictions, fear, and other such negative activities. Alternatively, we can use our energy to love, help out in the community and endeavor to do things that make ourselves and our neighbors better off.

Life is an adventure. It may not be the adventure you dreamed of, but it's still an adventure and there are many interesting things to do.

Our life paths will have ups and downs, mountains that must be climbed, abysses to avoid, bright times and darkness. Sometimes we will doubt ourselves and others. Occasionally, we will lose our way completely and have to find it again. But all of these difficulties will be easier if we choose to maintain a cheerful and willing attitude.

Besides the challenges of Parkinson's disease, Pat Hull survived three bouts of pancreatitis in 2004 that left her close to death, and she endures other health issues, too. Pat Hull continues to live life with zest and she still manages to keep up with Stanley.

CHAPTER THREE

KNOWLTON NASH

"Life is an ongoing mystery. What happens, will happen."

Knowlton Nash was diagnosed with Parkinson's disease in 2002. He is 79 years old.

My first exposure to journalism was selling newspapers for three cents at the corner of Bathurst Street and Eglinton Avenue in Toronto. The truck would drop off The Toronto Star and The Toronto Telegram in the afternoon and then, after school, I would open the bundles, take out the papers and stand on the street corner and sell them to passersby. I remember my biggest sales were on the day in June 1940 that Paris fell to the Germans. I had so many pennies in my pockets that my short pants almost fell off.

The first 'real job' I had was as editor of the Canadian High News. I then worked for British United Press, becoming Bureau Manager in Halifax, Vancouver and Toronto. I went to Washington in 1951 as Director of Information for the International Federation of Agricultural Producers *(IFAP).*

In that job I promoted world trade and the establishment of a world food bank to feed the world's hungry. I attended United Nations meetings, organized conferences and traveled to Europe and South America. Within about a year or so, I was writing articles for Maclean's magazine, the Financial Post, and various Canadian newspapers, as well as broadcasting for the Canadian Broadcasting Corporation *(CBC)*. I became the CBC Washington correspondent in 1958. I covered the Civil Rights Movement, the Vietnam War, and U.S. Presidents Eisenhower, Kennedy, Johnson and Nixon, as well as the assassinations of Martin Luther King and both Kennedys. I remained in Washington until 1969 when I returned to Canada and became Director of CBC News and Current Affairs.

Over my career as a correspondent, individuals have stood out in my mind more than events. The Kennedys—Bob and Jack—especially stood out for me. I had known them for a good long time because of my coverage of the Senate Labor Rackets Committee, when Bob was the Chief Counsel for the committee and Jack was a member of the Senate. They inspired hope in people and appealed to the better side of our nature. I had spent a good deal of time with them both personally and professionally so maybe I was biased.

Bob Kennedy would be my personal hero. He was soft-hearted but hard-headed. He had an extraordinary quality of caring and a deep commitment to make the world a better place. At times he could be a brass knuckle political street fighter and at times a rash romantic. Bob and Jack shared the same unrelenting competitiveness, but their styles were vividly different. Bob was more emotional, more intense, more impatient. Jack loved to gossip, Bob loved to argue. Jack was a pragmatist, Bob was an idealist.

I went with Bob on a campaign train in California a couple of days before his assassination and did one of the last long TV interviews that he gave. It was a challenging interview because he was in a very meditative mood. He was a fatalist and, with a sigh, he told me, "Look, fate is so fickle... life is a risk. You deal with what you have. You do what you can. But most of all you must try."

I also admired Mike Pearson tremendously (*Lester B. "Mike" Pearson was the Prime Minister of Canada from 1963-1968*). He was the quintessential nice Canadian. Ronald Reagan was a lot of fun to be with and I had a chance to have a couple of dinners with him when he was the Governor of California. It is always a challenge when someone you disagree with philosophically is a very nice person.

In 1978, I left my job as Director of News and Current Affairs to become anchor of The National (*CBC's nightly news program*) and the CBC Chief Correspondent. In the late 1980s, CBS in New York was anxious to lure away one of our best reporters and anchors, Peter Mansbridge. That would have been a devastating blow to the CBC and I wanted to keep Peter here in Canada working for the CBC. So, after a decade as anchor of the National, I decided to step down and let Peter take my place. I would host other programs and do documentaries. It was not a difficult transition at all because after leaving the role of anchor I was now so busy chasing news stories and doing various programs for CBC that I did not have much time to reflect on adjusting to doing something different. Certainly the CBC has benefited from the switch and I gained by having a slightly slower-paced, less frenzied existence.

My first sign of Parkinson's disease came while reading the newspaper. I noticed a slight tremor in my left hand when turning pages of The Globe and Mail one morning about five years ago. The tremor was more of a curiosity to me than anything else. I didn't mention it to the doctor for about a year. When I did, he made an appointment for me to go to a neurologist and I was diagnosed right away. I figured there were a lot worse things to be going through than living with Parkinson's, so I didn't feel too badly about the diagnosis. I think my basic nature is that when I am confronted with a challenge, I try to deal with it and then get on with life.

I have back pain at times, but probably my biggest frustration is not being able to speak more in public, which is too bad because I enjoyed talking to audiences. I can't do speeches now because my voice seizes up. Recently, I was the recipient of a couple of honorary degrees and lifetime achievement awards. I wrote the acceptance speeches and my wife delivered them. With my fingers dancing over the keyboard and her doing the talking, it worked out very well.

It's important to have a sunny outlook. I have always been an optimist about life in general. And I've been really fortunate to have had an exciting and enriching professional career doing something that not many people have a chance to do—and meeting, as the old cliché has it, so many interesting people. It's been a glorious way to make a living. I am even one who tends to respect politicians, and that is a rare breed in the business of journalism. I admire them and the sacrifices they make and, for the most part, I believe there are as many decent, honest politicians as there are journalists or teachers or any other profession.

I have been jogging since high school, although now I don't run too fast—it's more like plodding than jogging. While I used to run five to six miles, now I go out every morning and I do about three or four miles—jogging half and walking half. There is one advantage to having Parkinson's because I can now claim an extra five to ten strokes in my golf handicap.

I find myself tired a bit more, but I am not sure if that is a product of age or Parkinson's. There are a lot worse things that could be happening to you. With Parkinson's, you just have to cope with it and get on with it. In some ways, you don't feel as active as you used to. Maybe you are holding back the more exuberant members of your family sometimes. But you can't do anything about it so you might as well try to make the best of your day, of your night and your life.

Life is an ongoing mystery. What happens, will happen.

Knowlton Nash is one of the most recognized and best-loved media personalities in Canada. For ten years, he was the anchor of **The National.**

His career in journalism started in 1947 as a copy editor and reporter and, 60 years later, he is still working— writing a newspaper column for Osprey Media. Knowlton Nash is also the author of nine books.

CHAPTER FOUR

JOHN BALL

"Never again!"

John Ball was diagnosed with Parkinson's disease in 1983. He is 62 years old.

I was born in 1944, and grew up in a town called Lemon Grove, which is just to the east of San Diego. When we moved there, people were still herding cattle down the street in front of our house to graze them in the hills next to us. It was a semi-rural setting, but by the time I left there after high school it was all suburbia. Where the cattle had once grazed, there were now thousands of homes in their place.

I had always thought of myself as a runner. In high school, I ran a mile in just under four minutes and thirty seconds. In the 60s, that time would have won most of the state final track meets around the country, but it so happened that I couldn't even get out of my league finals because San Diego was a hotbed of running.

After college, I took flight training. I loved being a pilot and flying airplanes. I served as a medical evacuation pilot in Vietnam and was stationed in the Philippines during 1968 and 1969. We flew in and out of a bunch of places in Southeast Asia, usually rescuing or picking up people to take them to hospitals. It was nerve-wracking being shot at, and I felt badly for the flight nurses who were dealing with the wounded in the passenger section. There was a lot of stress associated with this type of flying.

Parkinson's symptoms started when I was 27, just a few years after I'd left Southeast Asia. First there was a spasm in my left foot, which I now know was dystonia. At the time, I just called it a cramp in my left foot. My toes would curl under whenever I tried to walk any distance on flat ground or when I got tired. As I think back on it, my exposure to Agent Orange while serving in Vietnam might have caused my Parkinson's.

As my mobility got worse over the years, I went from being an outfielder on my softball team to playing second base, then to being a pitcher and finally to playing as a catcher. I was reduced to the point that I couldn't even run to first base. They had to send a pinch runner for me if I actually got a hit. But one game, after taking a 'mystery tablet', I started throwing the ball back to the pitcher without having it bounce before getting to him. The pitcher came down off the mound and said, "John, what the heck is going on? You just threw the ball to me without it bouncing and you're standing up straight for the first time in years."

Out of frustration of not being able to figure out what I had, my doctor had given me some yellow tablets and said, "Take these. If they make any difference then we will have a better idea about what is causing your symptoms." I didn't think that was a good way to try and diagnose things, but for me it turned out to be a blessing in disguise when I took that first tablet before the softball game.

I went home that night and looked at the little packet of four or five tablets that my doctor had given me and then I read about them in my drug manual. It said the pills were Sinemet and that they were used in treating Parkinson's disease. I sort of figured out at that moment that what I had was Parkinson's. It was 1983, I was 39 years old, and I had been diagnosed almost by accident.

I felt better with this diagnosis because it actually allowed me to name and identify 'my enemy'. I was also excited because the Sinemet made me feel better than I had in years. For me, learning that I had Parkinson's was not a death sentence but a 'life sentence'.

At the time, I was working for American Honda. When I went back to the office the next day and said, "I've got Parkinson's disease," my boss replied, "Oh, is that what it is? Okay, get back to work." A year later, they promoted me to national manager of technical training. I eventually moved into a less stressful position as the Industry/Education coordinator for the company, which turned out to be a perfect role for me.

In 1996, at the age of 52, I decided that I wanted to run a marathon and I began training heavily for it. I succeeded in finishing it in just over four hours. The first words out of my mouth after completing it were, "Never again!" It took me a couple of hours to relax and realize what an accomplishment I had made. I had set a goal, trained for it and achieved it. I started to realize that there was a great deal more that could be accomplished by running a marathon. I could channel that energy to help other people as well.

One year, a group of us trained diligently for the Los Angeles (*LA*) Marathon and, on race day, we were joined by a couple of others who had not trained at our level but who wanted to run with us. We said OK but they were a bit slower than we were. After 19 miles of running, we had to decide if we should all stick together or if the group of us who had trained together should split away and try to break our time target. We decided that we were Team Parkinson and not 'Time' Parkinson so we all stuck together and finished six across at the finish line with our hands in the air.

I had run the LA Marathon for three years in a row when a friend of mine, Mary Yost, decided she was going to do it, too. Mary also has Parkinson's, and loves to stir things up. When she noticed the LA Marathon supported 50 charities in the community, she decided to find out if one of the Parkinson's organizations could be included. None of the national organizations had the time or personnel to put the effort together, so Mary called a meeting of nine individuals at her house in December 1999 and by March 2000, Team Parkinson was an official charity of the LA Marathon. In the first year we raised $50,000. In the second year, my wife took over being the chairperson and now my wife and I are co-chairpersons. It has become a year-round charitable effort to raise money for Parkinson's research. We are now the lead charity for both the LA Marathon and the San Francisco Marathon.

I look at Parkinson's as an obstacle to overcome, but Parkinson's is not a tragedy. Events happen in life, and we attach the meaning to those events and put our own stamp on things. The solution to problems comes from within yourself, not from outside. Only you can control your behavior. In running, people started breaking four-minute miles because they believed they could. Until something is done for the first time, nobody believes it is possible and, as with Parkinson's disease, the mind controls so much of what the body is capable of.

As you go through life, you learn how to make decisions, how to get support from people and how to use the resources available to you. In my 'toolkit' I have lots of resources, like my strength, my fitness and my training. Those are resources that I can draw on. I also have the knowledge and skills that I obtained through managing a department at work. I have a support system of my wife, my kids, my family and my friends. Parkinson's is merely an obstacle on the path. You need to use your own 'toolkit' to find a way over or around your obstacles. Don't give up on what you want to get done in life because you have Parkinson's.

Lack of success does not equal failure. When I look back at the things I have done, many have not worked. You can learn a lot by failing. Experiences that do not work may teach you enough so that you succeed the second time you try or you may learn that it is not something you want to pursue again. Either of these represents success, through both learning and failing.

Parkinson's has made me a better person and provided me with a chance to express myself in a different way. It is a blessing, not a curse. It has given me a way to meet some great people and to help others.

My goal in life is to help people with Parkinson's. That is what I've decided is going to satisfy my ultimate ambition in life, which is to leave the world a better place than I found it. It's like the simple rule that I learned in Boy Scouts which is, "Leave the campsite cleaner than you found it." If I can leave the world better than I found it, I will have done my job.

John Ball continues to be fully involved with Team Parkinson and is the author of a book called **Living Well, Running Hard.** *At the age of 62, he still runs marathons.*

CHAPTER FIVE

JANET SINKE

"You only get one shot at today."

Janet Sinke was diagnosed with Parkinson's disease in 2001. She is 56 years old.

Two years after I had been diagnosed with Parkinson's disease, I was sitting in my small office around three o'clock in the morning, reflecting on my newest little granddaughter. Then I started thinking about my two grandmas. I don't know why, but I vividly remembered details about them, like their hair and their voices. They were just the most wonderful women. I picked up a pen and I started to write. All the words came in rhyme and before I knew it, I had written my first book. It was called *I Wanna Go to Grandma's House* and it is about a young granddaughter who describes a fun-filled day with her grandmother. I wrote ten stories in eight weeks—it was like my brain was electric. One part of my brain was deteriorating, but the other part of my brain had gone off.

My daughters and my three daughters-in-law all work in education. They read the stories I had written and said, "Mom, these are really good! You've got to get these published." So I sent the first manuscript of *I Wanna Go to Grandma's House* to 54 publishing companies. I was rejected 54 times. I remember one rejection in particular that stated I needed more of a plot—that I needed to develop a story with problems. I decided not to follow their advice, and instead I kept the story upbeat, fun and sentimental with a concentration on the simple things in life. It is our bestseller.

I don't know if it was because I was aware that I had a deteriorating neurological disease or if it was because I was turning 50, but for some reason I didn't care about the rejections. I wasn't scared. I decided, "You know what? I'll do it myself." So I started my own company called My Grandma and Me Publishers. I knew nothing about publishing. I took that first year and spent over 12 to 14 hours a day just educating myself, getting books produced, and calling all over the United States. The first book was extremely well received and we sold 5,000 books in nine weeks. I got the books into the schools and things just snowballed from there. I wrote additional titles for the Grandma series and in less than three years 35,000 books have been sold. Had I not had Parkinson's, I doubt this would have happened.

I grew up on a farm in Michigan, where I went barefoot all my childhood. Ten of us living in a farmhouse—seven brothers and sisters and a mom and a dad—with only one bathroom. I shared a huge room on the top floor of the farmhouse with my other sisters and never had much privacy, which was fine. We never thought anything of it. But in spring, summer and fall, whenever I wanted to be by myself, I would go and sit in a big apple tree. I would plant my butt right where the branches came out—and I would read books and write different stories and reflections. As I got older, I worked on the school newspaper and I kept writing different things, but I would just kind of tuck them away. When I got out of high school, I did not pursue a career in writing but instead went to nursing school.

Tremors and other Parkinson's symptoms started in my mid-forties, but I just blew them off and ignored the fact they were occurring. In 1998, I began working at a brand new hospice that was designed for those who needed a place to spend their final days. I felt privileged to be part of a fantastic team of nurses and professionals who were smart, knowledgeable and fun. However, soon my balance started to deteriorate and the tremors got worse. I began to feel my voice going and people would tell me that they couldn't hear me when I was talking. My staff commented to me about how tiny my handwriting had become. I thought I had some arthritis in my hand. I could feel that I was moving slower and I couldn't keep up when I was walking with people.

In 2001, I went to the doctor and he looked at me and he told me that I had prominent masking features. It took him less than 30 seconds to diagnose me with Parkinson's. Around the same time, I was also diagnosed with celiac sprue disease, which is an intestinal malabsorption allergic-type reaction to wheat, barley, oats and rye.

After being diagnosed, I started to have other problems due to the malabsorption and Parkinson's, which ranged from night blindness to irregular heartbeats and anemia. It was a difficult time but luckily a new grandchild entered the picture. I helped to take care of her so my focus went away from myself. I thought to myself, "I am going to dance at her wedding, so I can't get down. I can't lie around. There is a lot to live for."

I was working full-time and I loved the work, but my family was very concerned about me because I had started collapsing at home, so I decided to step down from that position. Leaving full-time work was very difficult for me. I left the hospice in 2001, although I still occasionally help out part-time. I have now been working in the nursing field for over 35 years.

My husband and I have five kids who are all close together in age. The kids ended up starting families at the same time. Soon, we are going to have eleven grandbabies—the oldest one is five years old. It's great fun watching everything unfold. I just love being a grandma.

One night, I was kneeling on the floor, giving one of my granddaughters a bath and when I went to pick her up, I just kept falling into the tub before I managed to get her out. That scared me, so I called my doctor and I said, "You know I've got to do something. The drugs aren't working as well as they should." My worst fear is the possibility of dropping a grandchild.

My diagnosis could have been worse. I have looked after patients with brain tumors or other terminal diseases where the life expectancy is six months or less—witnessing their last days brings me back to reality. When I think of all the people whom I have cared for over the years, any number of them would give anything to change places with me.

I have been at the bedsides of hundreds of people who have died and no one talks about how big their house is or how much they have in their 401K or how fancy their car is.

People talk about things like relationships, baking bread, walking down dirt roads or other simple things.

Some days I move slower than I want and that is frustrating. Right now I probably take 20 pills a day. But in a way, getting Parkinson's has been one of my greatest blessings because it has given me an opportunity to look at life from a different mountain and to go down paths I would not have been on otherwise.

Try not to waste a day or an hour or even a moment of your life. Celebrate. Have fun. Enjoy the journey, for life is an exciting and holy adventure meant to be lived and embraced even in the darkest of hours. Look for blessings in the challenges that come along the way.

We, the Parkinson's population, still have a lot to give to others, despite the challenges and tough times we face with a deteriorating neurological condition. We all have gifts and love to give others. Every time that we help someone else there is a rippling effect that will assist others that we will never meet. When it comes our turn to leave this world, we will be remembered as people who made a difference.

You only get one shot at today. You will never live this day again so make it the best day you can.

Janet Sinke continues to write books and manage her publishing company. She has now published five books, the most recent being **Ten Lessons Learned.** *Janet Sinke still works part-time at the hospice, and also speaks publicly about her experiences with Parkinson's and publishing.*

CHAPTER SIX

RAUL YZAGUIRRE

"Parkinson's presents an opportunity to reflect on my life and to appreciate it more."

Raul Yzaguirre was diagnosed with Parkinson's disease in 1999. He is 67 years old.

I have had three major influences that have helped me tremendously, both in my life and in business. My maternal grandfather was an illiterate man who garnered the respect of everybody that he ever met. He was a very decent human being, and he taught me to do the right thing, to be happy, and to appreciate everything I have in my life. He taught me how to have a positive attitude and all about overcoming adversity in life.

Dr. Hector Garcia was the second major influence. He introduced me to the Hispanic and Mexican-American Civil Rights movement. He was a physician, and he founded the American GI Forum, which became the nation's largest

Hispanic veterans group. He believed in giving back and helping people.

The third person was John Gardner, whom I had a chance to work with for several decades. He had great involvement in public life. He was President of the Carnegie Corporation and also the Secretary of Health, Education, and Welfare under President Lyndon Johnson. He was my mentor—he motivated me to enter into public life and helped me to think through a lot of public policy issues. He had an ethic of service to others and of trying to make society better. I found him very inspirational.

When I took over the NCLR *(the National Council of La Raza is a Hispanic Civil Rights and advocacy organization)* in 1974, it did not have a vision or much momentum. The organization had been 'ground zero' for a lot of bickering and fighting that was ideological, philosophical and geographical. However, it had the right framework and it was definitely worth saving. Initially, we had to do a 'cleanup' operation and restructuring—which was very necessary at the time. I got the board of directors to think in terms of a larger operation with a goal, a vision of where we wanted to grow and develop, and to begin the practice of bringing additional talented people on board.

The 1970s were a high point for Hispanics—we were graduating a higher percentage of our young people from college and we were making gains in corporate employment and in other arenas. Since then, we have gone backwards—partly because we have been portrayed as being lawbreakers in terms of immigration. Now immigration issues suck up all the oxygen.

In 1999, I started to notice a twitching in my right thumb. I went to a neurosurgeon and he did a couple of MRIs and concluded that I had ruptured vertebrae in my neck. He said that was what was causing my twitching hand and that surgery would be the best option. Just prior to having the surgery, my doctor referred me to a neurologist, and the neurologist gave me the diagnosis that I had Parkinson's disease.

I was vaguely aware of what Parkinson's was. I had been in the Medical Corps while I was in the Air Force, and I knew that it was a degenerative disease. Many of the symptoms of the disease were familiar to me but more as theoretical issues, not on a personal level.

My symptoms have gotten steadily worse—my arm shakes almost all day long and my speech is getting a little more difficult to articulate—but my mind is clear and I am able to work. Some days are better than others—I have periods where I virtually forget that I have Parkinson's, and other days where it hits me hard.

I used to try to take advantage of almost every opportunity I had to communicate with the public. After the symptoms started to show more, I found myself not wanting to speak in public as much. There is a sense that you don't want to expose what you consider to be a weakness or a defect, which is why I now find myself asking my colleagues to speak for me at events or functions.

Now, when I speak to folks in public, I try to use humor. I start my speech by telling them that I have Parkinson's and that it is not a big deal, but that it does interfere with my drinking because my beer drinking hand has been affected—so now I spill a lot of beer. I find it relaxes me and also the audience and it allows them to focus on what I have to say and not my shaking hand.

Having a positive attitude is the most important thing. Parkinson's provides a new way to learn and to grow. It presents an opportunity to reflect on my life and to appreciate it more. It helps me focus on what I can do and what I cannot do. I feel lucky that I have Parkinson's now as opposed to 30 years ago, because at least there are options now with this disease whereas before there were not.

My biggest challenge is finding the time to do all the things that I want to do.

Raul Yzaguirre is a Civil Rights leader and was the President of the National Council of La Raza (NCLR), from 1974—2004. The NCLR is the largest national Hispanic Civil Rights and advocacy organization in the United States, helping more than 40 million Hispanics. The NCLR grew under his leadership—from nine employees to over one hundred—and it expanded to include not just Mexicans but also Puerto Ricans, Dominicans and others. The building for the NCLR headquarters in Washington, D.C. was renamed the Raul Yzaguirre Building in 2005.

Raul Yzaguirre is now the Presidential Professor of Practice in Community Development and Civil Rights at the University of Arizona.

CHAPTER SEVEN

LOUISE WHITNEY

"There are places a person with Parkinson's shouldn't be and this is definitely one of them."

Louise Whitney was diagnosed with Parkinson's disease in July 1997. She is 60 years old.

The first symptom I noticed was that my left arm didn't swing when I walked. I could still move it—so it wasn't paralyzed—but it just wouldn't swing naturally. A more annoying symptom occurred when I was driving—I would suddenly realize that all the muscles in my left leg had tightened up. I would relax the leg and the next thing I knew, it would be all stiff again. But it was the non-swinging arm that led me to visit my doctor. She concluded that I might have Parkinson's disease. I'd worked with people who had Parkinson's, so I was not surprised by her opinion. She sent me to a neurologist who confirmed the diagnosis. It was bing-bing-bing.

Prior to being diagnosed, my husband and I had decided to go to China for three to five years. My husband was with Eastman Kodak and he was offered an opportunity to help set up a new factory in Xiamen, which is a beautiful coastal city. I was leaving my professional career, my oldest son and his wife were expecting their first child, our youngest son was moving to Alaska and both of our parents were moving into smaller living quarters. I hardly even thought about Parkinson's because I had so many other things going on. The only thing I did do was ask the neurologist what he thought about the plan to go to China. He said, "Go for it."

China was a place I had never particularly wanted to visit, but it turned out to be just wonderful. The Chinese people were welcoming and gracious. Many of them were trying to learn English, so when we talked they would work on their English and we would practice our Chinese. We had taken lessons in Mandarin and we had tutors in the U.S. and China, yet still the Chinese had to work hard to understand us. Their language is a tonal one, which means you can say the same word with a different tone to it and it takes on a totally different meaning. For example, 'ma' can mean mother or horse.

We lived in an all-Chinese neighborhood, so when I went to the nearby market, I would somehow communicate through gestures and my basic Chinese, because the farmers in the market didn't speak any English. One day I went looking for chicken breasts but there were none on the counter and I couldn't remember how to say 'breasts'—so finally, in desperation, I grabbed my own to help get the point across. The farmer and his family dissolved into laughter, but immediately they knew what I needed. Every time after that, when I came into the market, they'd smile and laugh and hold up chicken breasts.

We traveled a great deal throughout China and Southeast Asia. Many of the places we visited required negotiating steep slopes or steps that were irregular in height and without railings. I was beginning to experience some balance problems and the grip in my left hand was weakening, but I refused to let that slow me down. On one occasion we were following a guide up a mountain path when the route entered a cave. It was dark, steep and narrow—and the hand and footholds were slippery. Suddenly I thought, "There are places a person with Parkinson's shouldn't be and this is definitely one of them." When I emerged on the other side I was triumphant that I had made it through.

While in China, we joined an adventure group from the Rochester area who were trekking for ten days through all the foothills of the Himalayan mountains of Nepal. Another couple we knew was also going and my husband really wanted to do it, too. I talked to the expedition leader who assured me that it was not a difficult trek and certainly doable. My neurologist said he didn't see why I couldn't do it. So I went—and I did it! One of my mantras has always been, 'It can be done and I can do it'. I don't know where I heard that the first time but, on the trek in Nepal, I would often say that to myself. For ten days we traveled on a path that took us up to where people live in the mountains, and also to a lot of Buddhist temples. I managed to keep up with everybody. We climbed ravines and slid down snow-covered fields. Sometimes I had to use a couple of walking sticks or hold onto somebody's arm, and when we stopped for lunch I usually fell asleep. But I did it. If I had known what it was going to be like ahead of time, I certainly never would have agreed to do it. But luckily, I didn't know that before the trek. It was an awesome experience. Proof that 'it can be done'.

I've now had Parkinson's for ten years. A big problem for me is what I call 'clognition'—I can't think quickly anymore, especially if I have several people talking or asking me for things at the same time. Fatigue is also an issue—my patience dwindles as I get tired which usually happens towards the end of the day. I have to plan my days around my energy level and sometimes allow for short naps.

The difficulties I encounter fastening jewelry clasps, folding t-shirts or ironing slacks irritate me. When I'm home alone I have sometimes resorted to pitching an uncooperative bracelet across the bedroom. I notice I have more of a tremor either when I'm nervous or when I'm tired. My gait is uneven at times and I have left-sided weakness. I now use a walking stick if I'm going to cross any large fields or walk any considerable distance.

It was these problems of fatigue and clognition that led me to resign from my job. It was a wrenching decision, and it made me see the disease in more vivid colors because it was progressing. I had been affiliated with Jewish Senior Life's Adult Day Services programs since 1981—as a social worker, director and a volunteer during the brief periods when I returned home from China. Leaving was very painful, but the progression of my Parkinson's disease gave me no choice.

I had some exposure to Parkinson's prior to my diagnosis because I had worked with patients who were mostly in the end stages of the disease. This knowledge helped finalize my decision to resign, because I don't know the course that the disease will take with me. I don't want to miss out on time with my husband, my children and my grandchildren, as well as time with my own mother.

I still ski, but not as frequently as I used to. I don't do the double black diamond runs anymore and actually I am moving towards skiing the green, easy slopes. I am involved with an exercise program designed here in Rochester specifically for people with Parkinson's disease. The program is run two days a week and I try to do it in between, but I have to admit that I'm not very faithful to the exercise regimen. I'm an avid creative writer but I can work at the computer only so long before my left fingers start punching in an extra 'e' or 'i' here and there. I love poking around flea markets but I need to brace my left arm, which aches if it is left to dangle. 'Shop till you drop' now means a couple of hours—not a whole day.

I often ask myself, "Do you have Parkinson's disease or does it have you?" There are aspects I cannot control, but there are also aspects that I can control. I used to be self-conscious about the tremors but I realized that they were not as significant to others as they were to me.

It is important to accept help and to ask for it when it is needed. I am still capable—I just need a little help along the way sometimes. Every now and then I talk to my friends about Parkinson's and that gives them the opportunity to ask me how things are going. I have great support from my husband, my family, and my friends. My husband has been my rock through this. He also gets frustrated by the changes in me. We are as open as we can be with one another, sharing our observations, concerns and feelings. We cry, we laugh, we hug and we go on. We attend monthly Parkinson's support group meetings where we have an opportunity to talk with and learn from other care partners.

I think it is key to remember that our worth as humans is not dependent on what we can do. We tend to think in terms of things like, "What did you get done this weekend?" Or, "What do you do for a living?" But that's not what is important. Our worth comes from just existing.

Louise Whitney is active in the Parkinson's Support Group of Upstate New York, serving on committees, and also editing the quarterly newsletter. As well, she is busy writing stories about her experiences in China.

CHAPTER EIGHT

BILL COMMANS

"My philosophy has always been the same—push the envelope."

Bill Commans was diagnosed with Parkinson's disease in June 2002. He is 76 years old.

My life has always been an adventure. Many times my wife told me that I lived on the edge of reason and exposed myself to risk. I spent my career as a chief engineer aboard ocean-going vessels—mostly oil tankers—and I've found myself in harm's way more times than I care to remember. Even my recreational interests were somewhat hazardous. While others might be happy on the golf course, I preferred downhill skiing and sailboat racing. Yet nothing I'd experienced in my life could have prepared me for the impact of Parkinson's disease.

I attended the New York State Maritime Academy and earned an engineering degree. I began working with Getty

Oil, and I eventually became the chief engineer on big ships such as oil tankers. When I first started working, the safety requirements were a great deal less stringent than today. At the time, they were very dangerous ships to be on, mainly because oil is an extremely volatile substance. The fire hazard is tremendous when 90 percent of the cargo is oil and gasoline. All in all, I spent over 20 years at sea.

Only recently have we become more aware of the side effects of asbestos and benzene, which are present on oil tankers. I was found to have some benign spots on my lung as a result of my exposure, and the spots are checked annually to ensure everything is OK. I speculate that exposure to these chemicals may have had something to do with my developing Parkinson's.

I first got married in 1960. My wife and I had two boys, who are now in their early forties. We were married 30 years before we divorced. I met my second wife in Toledo in 1991. I ended up marrying this wonderful lady, and we had ten lovely years together. It felt like the way a marriage should be—we communicated with each other wonderfully. Tragically, she passed away in August 2001.

My journey with Parkinson's began about five years ago during a routine visit to my doctor. I was feeling good and I was expecting to receive a clean bill of health. I told him that I was having more difficulty getting up from chairs, and getting in and out of cars. For me, this seemed to be a natural consequence of aging. However, the doctor looked more closely at me, and he recognized some of the classic symptoms of Parkinson's. He referred me to a neurologist who soon confirmed the diagnosis.

The combination of losing a loving wife and the onset of

Parkinson's drove me into a spin. I was not thinking straight. I didn't have anyone to help me and I had a house to contend with. I thought, "What will happen to me now? Why me?"

It seemed to me that the symptoms grew more severe virtually overnight. My writing became smaller and more difficult to read. My walking slowed to a snail's pace and I began dragging my left foot. The right side of my body became problematic and started to be almost inoperative. I had a lot of difficulty getting up from a seated position. I was disillusioned and feeling very sorry for myself. This feeling was compounded when three different types of medication failed to help. I felt defeated.

My outlook finally changed after I went to a Parkinson's conference in March 2003 and heard Janet Reno speak. I related to her discussion and she inspired me, because she had to deal with Parkinson's while being the Attorney General. After hearing her speak, I went on the Internet and aggressively read up on Parkinson's. It sometimes requires a great deal of research, but there are helpful answers to many questions on the Internet.

I concluded that there was no use in denying that I had it—the disease was not going to disappear. I chose to announce my ailment rather than hide it and I also learned to accept assistance from others. After I started to think about Parkinson's in a more positive way, I started to feel like I was taking control of 'my ship' again.

I realized that I needed help at home. Luckily, a lady who had occasionally been helping me, and who also had nursing experience, needed a place to stay. We came to an agreement and she became my 'caregiver'—a new term for me. She helped me with my walking, outfitted the house with safety equipment, and drove me everywhere I needed to go. I even resumed dining out, with her as my dinner companion. We were quite the odd couple, a petite younger woman and an old man, and we frequently drew attention, which I found quite humorous. One time, she was pulling me up from a restaurant chair and people were staring at us. With a smile, I remarked loud enough for everyone to hear, "This is the only way I can get her to put her arms around me!" She eventually left after four years as my caregiver, and I have since had difficulty finding a replacement.

I still have down or off periods but they are much less frequent. In my case, I believe the off periods happen when either I am eating poorly, experiencing stressful periods in my life, or consuming too much alcohol. I have learned that two drinks of anything is a definite limit and that my diet must be closely monitored. These are fairly easy factors to control. The stress of finances and living on a fixed income is more of a challenge.

Depression is something to be very aware of. I had a very bad scare while driving, and now I have to limit my driving. I gave in reluctantly and I was very depressed as a result of losing some of my independence. Luckily, I managed to get back on course with some help from others. If you are feeling down, make sure that you talk to someone you can trust and that you respect.

If you can laugh at yourself and your clumsiness and not curse every time you stumble, it makes things easier. The other day, I was walking the neighbor's toy poodle because the dog has taken a liking to me and actually prefers that I walk her instead of her owner. All was going well until the dog cut across my feet, and down I went! She then turned around and licked my face with an attitude like, "What are you doing on the ground?" You have to be able to laugh at things like that.

I am now living in Nashville, and I was invited to a conference hosted by the National Parkinson Foundation Center at Vanderbilt University in October 2005. The program included a speaker named Barbara Batson, an exercise guru who was interested in working with people with physical limitations. Her presentation inspired me to attend one of her aquatic classes. I was pleasantly surprised to find out how much variety, humor, singing, and laughing were included in her teaching. People were exercising, but they were also having fun. At first I was reserved, but the group finally got me to participate and now I loudly join in the singing—although I can't say my attempts to sing are anything more than just making noise. I also like talking to the other people in the class, and I always leave with a smile on my face. In a very short time, I felt an increase in my range of motion, which I directly attribute to the exercise.

I resumed playing card games like gin and cribbage, which are games that I had learned during the long hours when I was out at sea. Playing cards is a great way to keep the hands flexible. Shuffling is difficult but I can hold my own. I am also building ship and airplane models again, which is something that I have loved doing ever since I was ten years old. The first ones that I constructed were flawless but over the years the quality has slipped a little. My best job to date is a British Spitfire. I have since graduated to more complex ship models, which can be very challenging—especially when I am shaking like a leaf. Building models gives me peace and serenity.

I get frustrated sometimes by simple things like getting my pants on. One gets sick of hearing "One leg at a time." The correct answer in my opinion is "Any way you can." I usually have a down period at night. When I can't move, I just try to laugh and remind myself that I have Parkinson's and I can't do too much to get rid of it, so I might as well accept it.

I am convinced that my persistence in seeking out help and maintaining a positive attitude has made a powerful difference in my health. I also turn to God for comfort and hope. As an old saying goes, "Never give up, that's the secret to glory." Don't let Parkinson's get you down.

Don't ask for help unless you absolutely need it. Try to maintain your independence as much as possible. I can't clean floors or the house very well, but I do intend to maintain my independence on personal things. I think you need to be the 'captain' of your own medical program for it to be the most effective. I am steering my ship through difficult times.

My philosophy has always been the same—push the envelope. I have noticed that the people who seem to have the most positive attitude all have one thing in common—the drive to improve.

Bill Commans is currently involved in a clinical trial program and he continues to stay active—swimming or going to a gym twice a week, and walking whenever he gets a chance.

CHAPTER NINE

CHRIS OLSEN

"I started to panic, thinking I was having a heart attack."

Chris Olsen was diagnosed with Parkinson's disease in 2004. She is 58 years old.

I wanted to be a mapmaker, so I went to study cartography at Camosun College just outside Victoria, British Columbia. I was always interested in geography and drawing so I thought cartography would be a great fit because it required very detailed hand drawing. However, the only jobs available after I finished the course were in camps that were in remote areas of northern British Columbia. This meant that I would have to sleep in the same rooms with, and use the same showers as the men because the camps would not have separate facilities. I wasn't prepared to do that, so I switched from cartography to graphic arts and eventually settled into a career in the book publishing industry.

My first noticeable Parkinson's symptoms occurred in September 2003, roughly one year before I was diagnosed.

I thought I had a pinched nerve perhaps, but I did not think much about it as I figured it was as a result of sports injuries that I had incurred before. Then a small tremor I had in my right hand began to get worse. I was also starting to suffer from extreme tiredness. I was officially diagnosed with Parkinson's disease in September 2004.

My reaction was one of shock and despair. I knew nothing about Parkinson's and so I was fearful and I didn't know what to expect. After reading Michael J. Fox's book and learning about his experiences, I was struck by how similarly my symptoms played out. I had always taken care of myself, I was physically active and I was a vegetarian—I could not understand why I would get something like this.

One night, I felt a very heavy sensation on my chest. I was getting short of breath and I could not move. I started to panic, thinking I was having a heart attack. My husband and I didn't call 911 because there was no reason why I should be having a heart attack. Instead, we called the University of British Columbia health hotline and it turned out that I was having a panic attack. I have learned how to cope with panic attacks through deep breathing and by changing what I am doing. For example, now if I feel one coming on, I take the dog for a walk to distract myself.

After being told I had Parkinson's, one of the first things I did was call my boss and tell her my diagnosis. She said, "Come to work when you are ready. We are fully prepared to work with you and your symptoms. We will change your workspace and do whatever you need." I only took off a couple of days and then I picked myself up and went back to work. I did not look back and have continued to work full-time.

I had a few times when I needed to go for a walk and cry, but eventually I just started to accept how things were. I have some 'off' days, but my co-workers have learned to understand my symptoms. My job requires me to do tons of data entry. I am slower than I used to be because now I have to use my left hand instead of my right hand to do a lot of the work. Co-workers also talked to me about Parkinson's and asked me how I was doing and if there had been any breakthroughs in research or whatever. I really appreciated this as it made me feel like I did not have to hide anything.

My husband and I both cried when we found out that I had Parkinson's—and then we decided to do what we could. When I was weak he was strong. I could not have asked for a better person to go through this with—he has been my rock. My two children and one granddaughter are also supportive and understanding. I also draw strength from my mom, who is 82 and has bad arthritis in her hip and knee. She has a dog and takes it for a walk three times a day, hobbling with her cane. She's like the Energizer Bunny— she just keeps on going.

I used to be self-conscious and hide my hand in my pocket or behind my back so that no one would see my shaking, but now I do not care as much if people see that. When I recently went through my neighborhood to collect pledges for a Parkinson's walk many people were surprised to learn that I had it.

It takes me longer to get dressed now and I have to get up a little earlier to get organized for work. I have joined a fitness club and they are very good at finding ways for me to exercise and get around the things I cannot do. I want to work full-time until I am 65 or, if necessary, scale back a bit in a few years. One concern I have is that I don't know what to expect for the future, as Parkinson's plays out differently for everyone. Hopefully I will be fine and find new ways to cope with the progression of Parkinson's.

The first thing I see in the mornings is the mountains, and as the year goes on and it gets colder it is exhilarating to see the snow accumulate on them. I eat my lunch by the Fraser River in the heart of Vancouver, watching seals and kingfishers. My husband and I walk almost every day after dinner. Some days we walk slowly with our dog, an American Eskimo called Toka. Other days we walk with purpose, depending on the stresses of our working day. We like to walk through many places, like Stanley Park or in Richmond on paths where we can watch eagles and see them with their eaglets, or observe herons and owls. In the west end of Vancouver, there is a seawall where we can walk by the ocean. It is beautiful. Every day I am grateful to live here in British Columbia.

I have changed quite a bit since being diagnosed. I am far more peaceful in my life and with my being. I now cope better with all the things that used to stress me out. It is not worth getting upset over little things. I think it is a good change. I have also begun to explore various spiritual avenues and I am thinking more about life in general.

I don't want to put people in a position where they might be uncomfortable with my disease. I don't feel sorry for myself or worry or lament, "Why me?" Parkinson's is debilitating and life altering, but I am able to arrange my life so that I can get more from it. I have people that I am responsible for and things I want to do before my life is over. I can still do a lot of things—just a bit slower than before.

A friend of ours who was a quadriplegic recently passed

away, and he had always believed in surrounding himself with positive people doing positive things. I believe the positive things are there—you just have to look for them. I try to keep laughter close to the surface—I think we all need to find the humor that is around us.

Don't withdraw into yourself. Keep active and find a reason to get up in the morning.

Chris Olsen and her husband are baseball fans and in the upcoming years they aim to visit every baseball park in North America.

CHAPTER TEN

IRV POPKIN

"It felt like I had won both an Academy Award and also scored the winning touchdown in the Super Bowl."

Irv Popkin was diagnosed with Parkinson's disease in 1989. He is 74 years old.

I grew up in Pittsburgh and, after graduating from high school, immediately went to work because we were poor. My mother was partially blind and unable to work and my father had died of leukemia when I was four years old. He had been gassed in the First World War and this may have played a role in his developing leukemia. I was in the Army from 1953 to 1955 and, after being honorably discharged, I went to the University of Pittsburgh and studied journalism.

After graduating, I looked for jobs in advertising. The best one I could get was only paying $65 a week. I was already making $65 per <u>night</u> selling encyclopedias so I decided to pass on the advertising job. To sell one set of encyclopedias,

I needed to knock on 50 doors. Going door to door in the evenings, I found out that husbands and wives would rarely be together—I had to have both spouses together to do a presentation. Of the 50 doors I knocked on, 25 would have no answer and 20 would have only one spouse at home. The remaining five doors that I knocked on had both spouses at home. I would always ask them, "If you owned a set of encyclopedias, would they be used and appreciated?" If the couple answered "Yes" then I would continue trying to sell them. On average, I would make two presentations a night and usually close one of the two—which made for a very nice living. I was in the encyclopedia business for ten years and even won a Cadillac for high sales. Eventually, I became a national sales trainer for the company.

I started to notice the first symptoms of Parkinson's disease when I warmed up for a handball match and my left side started to shake. I was 57 when I was diagnosed with Parkinson's. I had an excellent doctor and he sent me to the University of Pittsburgh Medical School. They put me on Levodopa, which gave me a new life. I became strong and had no shaking. My energy returned as long as my medication was kicking in. I continued playing handball for five years but eventually I started to fall during games because I couldn't change directions. I finally gave up handball when my back started to go and I couldn't make the quick adjustments in order to play competitively.

Believe it or not, I was never depressed upon hearing I had Parkinson's—why I will never know. Probably because I have a positive nature. In my opinion, the worst fear is the fear of the unknown, so I read everything I could and eliminated my concerns. I concluded that I had at least ten good years before I might be in a wheelchair. I asked myself if I could face that possibility and I decided that I could. Luckily, I am still not in a wheelchair.

After being diagnosed with Parkinson's, I decided to enter the insurance business. It was something that I could do part-time, which was a better fit with my energy and stamina. When I sold insurance, I was upfront with people about the reasons for my shaking so that they would not think I was nervous by the time I got to the point of trying to close the sale.

I do have minor frustrations trying to do simple things like buttoning my shirt or tying my shoes. My biggest challenge was the side effects of the Levodopa, which gave me horrible dyskinesia that often made people very uncomfortable. Kids sometimes would stop and stare at me when I walked. I would go into the same Wendy's restaurant frequently, and after a while the staff would all pick the cups off the tables when I walked in. Once I was in a bagel shop just reading the paper, and then all of a sudden my foot kicked out and I sent a chair flying across the middle of the shop. My medications have been a tremendous help. I am blessed that I live in an age where there have been great improvements in medicine—my dyskinesia now is not as bad as it once was.

I continued to exercise and walk on a track in my funny way, with my right leg way out in a Groucho Marx-like walk. One day, I got tired of this so I decided to see if I could run with my limp. Once I started to run all my symptoms disappeared—I could run just as fast and gracefully as I did before Parkinson's appeared.

My wife believes in tough love—she does not feel sorry for me but she does excuse some things. For instance, I never was neat but now I am even messier, so she picks up after me. We have been married 47 years. I am lucky to have a great family with two children and three grandchildren. My family and friends treat me the same and they do not view me as being sick—just slowing down.

Getting involved in a support group is definitely one of the important things to do in my opinion. I didn't attend any support group events until ten years ago, when a friend persuaded me to go to a meeting. The food was good and I saw that people were doing pretty well and not feeling sorry for themselves, which was great considering how long some of them had been living with Parkinson's. They kept inviting me back so I continued to go to the meetings.

One of the things I believe is that one should keep busy helping others because it makes you feel good about yourself. I have taken great joy from some of the meetings and things we have done with the support groups. For instance, we created the fundraising idea of a fantasy walk that would also allow people in wheelchairs or with limitations to be able to participate. The fantasy walk takes place in the imagination of the Parkinson's patients, their families and their friends, as they travel in their minds to exotic locations. We have walked on the Great Wall of China, strolled the beach of Maui, climbed Mount Everest, bounced on the moon, and even shrunk ourselves in size so that we could walk through the human brain.

I hate to ask people for money, and I especially hate when people say "No." To get around this, we wrote letters, describing the fantasy walk in detail, and then we each mailed 20 of these letters to people who knew us. For the Great Wall of China, we wrote about what it was like walking up the hill and seeing mountains and then we included pictures of the mountains. At the start of the letter we would write, "Close your eyes and visualize" and at the end of the letter we would write, "Now open your eyes and walk over to your checkbook." We usually get about 70% of our letters returned with donations!

When I found out that I had won the 2005 John Heinz community service award for my volunteer work, I was humbled because there were many other worthy nominees who were terrific people. I felt like I had won both an Academy Award and had also scored the winning touchdown in the Super Bowl.

I think it is important to not self-obsess. You need to smile and snap out of it. I like to make people laugh and I even wrote some jokes for a book called *Parkinson's Can Be Fun*. You won't go wrong if you exercise, eat well, and keep a positive attitude.

My hope is to see the fundraising component of the support group eliminated—because it would mean that we would have finally found a cure for Parkinson's.

Irv Popkin was selected from among 45 nominees to receive the 2005 John Heinz community service award for his volunteerism. The award is given annually by the Alexis de Tocqueville Society of the United Way of Allegheny County, Pennsylvania.

Irv Popkin is a leader of South Hills Parkinson's Support Group, which is better known as the 'Movers and Shakers'.

CHAPTER ELEVEN

MARGARET HANSELL

"Boy, if you have to have a disease, you sure have an interesting one!"

Margaret Hansell was diagnosed with Parkinson's disease in 1975. She is 62 years old.

I fell in love with my future husband, Allan Hansell, in 1962. We met during the second week of college—we were at Earlham College in Indiana where I was majoring in history—and we dated for four years before marrying two weeks after we graduated. Our son was born in 1968 and we had a daughter in 1970. In August of 1972, Allan landed a faculty position teaching in the biology department at Saint Mary's College of California so we moved out west and have been in the San Francisco Bay Area ever since.

I loved spending time with our children, as well as reading, sewing or cooking. I was a full-time mother and president of a nursery school co-op. As a family, we liked to camp and backpack and have had the excitement of encountering scorpions and bears. Frequently, we took several cars of college students with us and we would drive off in caravan style and get ourselves into all sorts of messes, like getting bogged down in sand dunes. We had great fun on our adventures.

In 1975, my hands started to get stiff. I thought it was stress and I would shake out my hand but the stiffness would not go away. I started to notice that my hand would not move properly when I did simple tasks like scrambling eggs, waving good-bye or writing. Then my toes began cramping under my right foot and it got to the point where I could run better than I could walk.

By the end of the year, I was getting kind of concerned, so my doctor set me up with a neurologist. I was easily diagnosed because, unbeknownst to me, my right arm was not swinging. When I walked across the room in front of the neurologist, it was obvious to him. He said, "I am sorry to tell you this, but you have a degenerative disease. However, there are a lot of new drugs in the pipeline and the future is looking very positive. When you get to the point where you need them, the drugs should be all ready for you." I kept thinking, "What is the name of the disease? What is it? Say it!" He told me that the name of the disease was Parkinson's. I was 30 years old.

My doctor gave me the contact number for a local group, but at the time there was no information available for young-onset or newly-diagnosed people. I was more puzzled about the disease than upset—at that point, I didn't even know what anyone looked like who had Parkinson's. When Allan came home, I told him what I had and he was not familiar with it either. So he went to the library and when he returned he came bounding into the house and said, "Boy, if you have to have a disease, you sure have an interesting one!" That's what you get for marrying a biologist!

I did learn that I had a few contributing risk factors for Parkinson's. I grew up in a polluted industrial town in New Jersey that used pesticides. The town had a heavy mosquito abatement program—with fog-like sprays that we loved to run through as kids. An artesian well served as the source for the town's drinking water. Not long after I was diagnosed, my 60-year-old mother was told she had Parkinson's, too.

I had written my Law School Admissions Test prior to being diagnosed and I resolved not to let Parkinson's stop me from becoming a lawyer. I went to Golden Gate University in San Francisco, which is known for its evening programs. The night schedule worked well, because I had kids in nursery school and kindergarten. I became a lawyer in 1981 and practiced for about four years.

During the 1984-85 school year, Allan went on sabbatical. I closed my family law practice and we went east. Allan collapsed going across the country and when we got to Maryland, where he was to do research at the Institute of National Health, he had to have a quintuple bypass. He was only 40 years old. I felt we were both too young to have his heart problems and my Parkinson's. Luckily he recovered in grand fashion and we had a glorious year on sabbatical.

We moved back to the West Coast the next year and I started to experience 'on and off' times. I had planned to go back to work, but I just could not function well enough to manage a law practice. Legal insurance became prohibitive because I was not working full-time. And you know, you cannot tell a judge, "Your honor, I am having an 'off' time. Could we stop the trial?"

The hardest thing for me was accepting limitations and cutting back on my hopes and dreams. I used to love rock climbing, but I had to give it up shortly after I started law school. I just didn't trust my body anymore. I fall a lot now, which upsets me, but I still manage to get along. I get so tired of it—so once in a while I let loose with a primal scream, which helps. I have probably taken every medicine that has been on the market, at one point or another.

Allan has been marvelous. With his love and support, I came to accept that I was still the same person that I had been prior to diagnosis. We have always talked about Parkinson's with our kids. They are comfortable discussing it and they like to tease me in fun fashion. I used to be called the 'Cardboard Mommy' because I was so stiff. We also had the 'Society of silly walkers'. It was similar to the Monty Python television show skit about silly walking, except with us it was the 'Hansell silly walkers' and every time I began walking funny they would all imitate me. It was a hoot and a howl.

In the late 80s, I became involved with a support group and also with the Parkinson's movement and lobbying on a national and state level. I am proud of the overall spirit that our chapter has, as well as seeing the chapter growing, reaching out and putting on programs.

Another thing that has helped me is taking on new activities and interests instead of focusing on things that Parkinson's prevents me from doing. I love birdwatching and, although I can no longer participate in the hikes that are necessary to find some of the most sought-after birds, I can watch slide shows put on by those lucky enough to see them. I have replaced walking on trails with moving along on a little electric scooter where the trail permits. I can also get involved in issues involving questions of local, state and national importance which affect birds, so that our children can still enjoy them in the future. As well, I can still write letters with my thoughts about Parkinson's issues to congressmen!

I started a singing group and we call ourselves the 'Tremble Clefs'. I think the concept originated in Phoenix about five years ago. I loved the idea, and I got a grant from the National Parkinson Foundation and started a group out here. We are a collection of caregivers, family members and patients who all get together and sing. It is open to anyone connected with Parkinson's. Anyone can sing—and you do not have to sing well! It is good exercise for the voice quality, too. About 14 to 18 of us meet once a week, and we are doing gigs about every month and a half. We sing all the old-fashioned kinds of songs, like *Downtown, When The Saints Go Marching In*, various African melodies, and *Give My Regards To Broadway*. We are having a ball doing it.

Allan and I recently went on a trip to Russia. We flew from Moscow for ten hours to the middle of Siberia, and then we took the trans-Russian railroad to Lake Baikal. We were on the train for two nights and three days. Prior to the trip, I thought Siberia was all deep dark woods and pine forest. But instead, it was rolling farmland with little towns dotted along the way. Sometimes the train would stop along the track and we would get out and pick flowers. I was terrified that my pills would be taken away from me—worrying about that possibility created huge anxiety. I don't really know how I got through the trip, but I did.

One of my keys to success has been the benefits of a twice-weekly exercise class with a group of other Parkinson's patients. My muscles and bones stay toned up and I generally feel much better after a class. There are many forms that exercise can take—from yoga to swimming. One thing you find out as you get older is that not all problems are because of Parkinson's disease. It is very important to keep active.

I think it is also helpful to get involved with groups or organizations. Support groups have a variety of resources available to assist you with everything from housing to neurologists. I am a firm believer in sharing experiences and helping others who are in the same situation.

Regardless of your situation, there are still lots of things that you can do or look forward to doing.

Besides being an avid birdwatcher, Margaret Hansell is currently in the process of editing an autobiography of her father who was a minister, professor and heavily involved in the development of assisted living facilities.

CHAPTER TWELVE

STEVE BOHANNON

"If we do not feel like it, we are going to do it anyway!"

Steve Bohannon was diagnosed with Parkinson's disease in 1999. He is 58 years old.

I first noticed something was not right when I went to a high school open house and I could not pick up papers off a table. I used to travel on business trips and my muscles would get all knotted up. I would try to stretch and move, but sometimes even walking would get difficult. It was about three years from the onset of these symptoms until early December 1999, when I officially found out that I had Parkinson's.

My dad had Parkinson's, too. He was diagnosed at the same age that I was—50 years old. He had it for 23 years before he passed away in 1989, ten years prior to my being diagnosed. My Parkinson's presents itself much differently than my dad's did. I have rigidity, limited facial expression and difficulties with speech, whereas my dad had a big tremor. My dad was in the food processing business, so we grew up living in a lot of agricultural areas that likely had exposure to pesticides. I speculate that this might have been a contributing factor to my father and me getting Parkinson's.

After being diagnosed with Parkinson's I was sad—then angry—but I went through these emotions very quickly. I have always been a positive person, and my dad was always very positive, too. He used to send me motivational books and pamphlets on a variety of subjects. After a couple of months I accepted the hand that I was dealt.

Between school terms at university, I worked at General Mills. Upon completing my Master's in Business, I returned there to work full-time. After being diagnosed, I let my managers know but I asked them not to tell others. I tried to hide my Parkinson's from my co-workers, but people could see something was wrong and they started to treat me differently. It was certainly a lesson in humility, and I thought about how some people have to endure their whole life being a little different. I found out that it was better when I explained what was going on to all my co-workers because they were very positive and good to me once they understood my situation. I retired at age 55 after working there for a total of 33 years.

My family has always been very important to me. My wife and I married in 1981 and we have five wonderful children, aged 18, 22, 24, 35 and 37. The two oldest are stepchildren. I miss the family trips we used to take. We would go to the seaside in Oregon and play on the beach, building sandcastles and jumping in the crashing waves. I loved the smell of salt water and the seaweed washed up on the shore. At night we would make a crackling fire on the beach and I would tell the kids stories.

I spend a lot on my kids. I just cannot say no to them. For example, when I go shopping with my daughter, if she sees something she wants, I just buy it. I bought all my kids second-hand cars this year. I need to stop it. There is a side effect with some Parkinson's meds that leads to behavior like compulsive gambling. I don't have the gambling problem but I do have a compulsive behavior issue. I was recently advised to slow down on what I give my kids, or I would spend my retirement savings and face serious financial consequences.

Parkinson's can definitely affect relationships. I think it is important to understand that people around you need time away. I try to encourage my family to take breaks—it can be tiring for them to be around me.

I am a Type A personality, and I have had to learn to accept getting two or three things done in a day and not ten. My medicine frequently gives me temporary brain clog. When that happens, I just wait for it to pass and then try to get some tasks done. I have learned that it is better to accept it than to fight it.

I am getting close to the maximum of how many meds I can take. I have trouble when a doctor says, "This is the best I can do for you." I have tried many different approaches and have even switched neurologists. I am currently having a real challenge sleeping because I have changed my meds. I used to gradually come down off my meds, but now it is like falling off a cliff. I have talked to my doctor and we hope to solve this. I never give up.

I have always liked the outdoors. I play tennis, go hiking and

I like to ride my bike. I used to be on the golf team in high school but golf is too time-consuming for me now and so tennis has become my favorite sport. I love a long rally where I am gasping for breath at the end of it. Tennis is a terrific workout, and whether or not I win doesn't matter to me. Sometimes playing tennis is easier than walking and it forces me to stretch, which feels great. Exercise is one way that I can get myself through or out of a difficult time. Instead of curling up in a corner and feeling depressed, I take a long walk, lift weights, play tennis or get on an exercise machine. Whenever I do this, I always feel much better.

You need to keep active mentally, too. I am very excited about an invention that I have been working on for a couple of years. It seems like things are falling into place. I think there is a definite tie between Parkinson's disease and creativity. I had never written poetry before Parkinson's, but now I like to write it. One of my favorite poems that I have composed is called *Declaration 2005*, and it is about not giving in to Parkinson's. The part of it that summarizes my outlook reads: "If we do not feel like it, we are going to do it anyway! No longer are we going to miss all the activities that we did yesterday."

Recently I've started to put the stories I used to tell my kids into writing. They quickly became a series of books called *All Of A Sudden*, where kids go from reality to fantasy and back. I am hoping to get them published. Writing is a huge release for me, and I am not sure that I would have done any of this if I did not have Parkinson's and a bit more time to reflect.

There is a huge economic benefit to this country for finding a cure for Parkinson's and other related diseases. We need to cut through the politics that goes with stem cell research.

I believe that a cure for one neurological disorder would lead to other cures. I wish there was more collaboration in research. I read research from all countries, including China and India. If there was some interesting breakthrough in another country and if the research looked positive, I would get my doctor's opinion and then jump on an airplane if necessary to investigate it further.

We should communicate to friends and family that, while we want to maintain our independence as much as possible, we might need their help a little more than we did in the past. We also have to be able to ask for assistance in a way where we do not give up our dignity. We still need their love and support and it is important for our family and friends to know that our self-worth probably could use a little more reinforcement than normal.

There are many situations that could be much worse to deal with, and you do not have to look far to see that. My family and my faith have given me the strength to get through difficult times, and my sense of humor has helped me, too. I feel strongly that there is a cure on the horizon, and for a lot of diseases that cannot be said. I consider myself lucky because I am young enough that I feel I will have many Parkinson's-free years ahead of me when the cure is discovered.

Every significant accomplishment or discovery starts with a dream. Never stop dreaming.

Steve Bohannon continues to write poetry and books and to work on his invention.

CHAPTER THIRTEEN

SHELBY HAYTER

"26 miles for Boston—one cure for Parkinson's."

Shelby Hayter was diagnosed with Parkinson's disease in March 2005. She is 42 years old.

I was always active. I liked playing outdoor sports like softball, soccer and tennis, and going cross-country skiing. When I was 16 years old, I wanted to challenge myself because I had been competing in running races since grade seven, so I ran in the Toronto Marathon. My goal was just to finish it. I completed it in three hours and thirty minutes.

I married an Air Force boy a few weeks after I graduated from teachers college and we immediately moved out to Moose Jaw, Saskatchewan. It was a new adventure and an awful lot of fun. The military had us move five times in the first ten years. We lived in Saskatchewan, Nova Scotia and Ontario. We lived by the seat of our pants, because our plans could change at any moment if my husband had to leave for a few days. I learned to be totally flexible and to always have a 'Plan B'.

My younger sister Andrea had a lifelong goal to run in the Boston Marathon. I decided that I would also run in Boston so that we could do the race together. To qualify for the Boston Marathon, you have to complete a 26 mile marathon in a set time based on your age and gender. I qualified by running the 2004 Toronto Marathon and my sister achieved the qualifying time in a subsequent marathon.

Around October 2004, I started to feel as if I had a one-pound weight on my left side while I was running. I decided to investigate the cause, mainly because Andrea had survived a brain tumor and I also had an aunt and a grandma with Parkinson's. I had three young children at the time, and I was not going to push myself over the barrier in my training for Boston if I was dealing with a major health issue.

That same month, I saw my family doctor and she put me through all of these tests, like CAT scans, MRIs, and blood tests. I tested negative on everything. But then a friend of mine told me she noticed that my left hand was not swinging like the right one was. I had no idea that had been happening. Also, when I had my head on my pillow at night, I could feel my left hand through the pillow. It felt like my hand had the faintest movement—sort of like a car idling. In February 2005, I was skiing with a friend who was a nurse and I described to her how sometimes, when I was washing my hair or typing on the computer, my left hand did not work as well as my right hand did. She recommended that I get a second opinion. One month later I went to a different neurologist, who diagnosed me with Parkinson's.

I knew that my grandma kind of shook but that was basically

about the sum of my knowledge regarding Parkinson's. I accepted the diagnosis immediately and I told the neurologist, "I am training for a marathon—what are your thoughts on this?" He said to keep an eye on things, but that if I was feeling OK, then I should go for it. That was the green light that I needed.

I was diagnosed late on a Friday afternoon. On Saturday morning, I went for a run and I thought to myself, "I have a lot of friends and family who will want to do something to support me." I thought that maybe I could design a family fun day or a picnic day in the park. Then I thought, "What are the chances that someone would be diagnosed with Parkinson's one month before they were to run the Boston Marathon?" When I finished my run, I went inside our house and asked my husband, "What if I ran in the Boston Marathon and we devised a slogan and I tried raising money for Parkinson's?" He loved the idea immediately, which inspired me to put it into action.

On Monday, my husband and I walked into the office of the Parkinson Society Ottawa *(PSO)* office. They were stunned to hear my story. They had been trying to decide who would be their new spokesperson and what the theme would be for Parkinson's Awareness Month. The PSO decided to have me as their spokesperson because I was a young-onset Parkinson's patient with a unique story. We gathered media attention with the fundraising slogan, "26 miles for Boston—one cure for Parkinson's." The story took off! I had thought that my friends, family, and neighbors would help—which they all did—but the support went way beyond anything I could have imagined. It was like a 'small town story' where checks were being handed to me left, right and center and online donations were being completed or called in over the phone.

The Boston Marathon starts in a tiny town called Hopkinton, which is 26 miles outside of Boston. Twenty thousand people qualified for it, so we had to be bussed into the area where the race starts, because it was so crowded. It was beautiful, sunny and 70 degrees on the day of the race. We were there about two hours before the race, and people were eating, drinking fluids, massaging, and warming up while bands were playing. Each racer wears a bib that has a number on it denoting where they start the race—faster qualifying times start at the front. My sister and I were in the middle in a corral with others who had qualified with the same times. When the starting gun went off, it took us something like five or ten minutes just to get to the starting line.

The race was run on Patriots Day which, in 2005, occurred on April 18. We were running over hill and dale and on all kinds of country roads from small town to small town. Patriots Day is a holiday in the state of Massachusetts, so there were a lot of people sitting on lawn chairs and having picnics. It was a big event, and the route was crammed with thousands of people, sometimes three or four rows deep, partying, watching and cheering, and passing you juices and drinks. I saw families, motorcycle gangs and, when we went by fire stations, they even had the hoses out to cool things off. We ran by a college and girls from the dorm rooms were all hanging on the gates cheering and high-fiving the runners. If a runner couldn't manage the race physically, they would still get pulled along just from the energy of the crowd. I felt like I was running on clouds. I completed the race and we ended up raising in excess of $36,000 for Parkinson's research.

I still teach elementary school children, now as a supply teacher. The young ones are very cute and they are completely comfortable asking me questions. One little girl came up to me and asked, "Do you still have Parkinson's?" I told her that I did and she replied, "But the Boston run is over!"

Another time, I went to a cross-country running meet as a parent-volunteer, and this little nine-year-old girl was tying up her shoes to get ready for a race. She looked up at me and asked innocently, "Have they found a cure yet?" I replied, "Oh no, not yet." She looked back and literally stared at me for a moment and then she shook her head in disgust before going back to tying her shoes.

I am so fortunate. I am sure that some people look at me and think, "What a shame, she is so young and she has young children,"—but, my goodness me, when you have to take care of children you cannot focus or dwell on yourself. With children, you have to sit and practice piano with them, take care of their sore knees, tie their shoes, take them to soccer practice, or help them with their homework. It is an absolute blessing to have children because they ground you. Children are a huge distraction in a very positive way.

We all have to deal with situations in which we don't have control over the outcome. But we can control how we mentally deal with the situation. Getting involved in a young-onset support group has helped me because I can learn, take notes, and get comfort from people in the same situation. I strongly believe the key is to focus on what you can do, because that is a positive approach, as opposed to dwelling on what you can't do.

One thing that I can do is to use my energy and enthusiasm to help raise money for research and also to create awareness about the disease.

Shelby Hayter has created a program for the school system in Ottawa called **Pass the Baton for Parkinson's.** *The program aims to increase awareness of Parkinson's disease and to raise funds to help find a cure. The message of* **Pass the Baton for Parkinson's** *is that it takes teamwork among patients, neurologists and researchers to help find a cure. The program is expanding and has had successful results in only its second year.*

CHAPTER FOURTEEN

JOHN THOMAS

"My wife put the needle into my arm and gave me a shot. In about five minutes I got out of the wheelchair."

John Thomas was diagnosed with Parkinson's disease in 1983. He is 70 years old.

One night my wife, who was a nurse, noticed my fingers shaking at the supper table. She told me that I should go see our family doctor, so I went to see him and he referred me to a neurologist who diagnosed me with Parkinson's. I was 46 at the time. I only knew what he had told me about Parkinson's. He mentioned the fact that a lot of people have it, but they don't know it or it doesn't bother them. They can live a normal life without medication, and every once in a while they shake a little bit. That made me feel better and put me at ease knowing that people with Parkinson's usually have no other problems.

He was obviously very wrong...

I was born in Canonsburg, Pennsylvania in 1937. Shortly after high school, I went into the Navy and was on a submarine from 1956 to 1960—we were stationed in Norfolk, Virginia. I got married soon after getting out of the service and one week after our wedding, I started working with Columbia Gas. I planned to stay with them until I was 55 years old.

For the first 15 years at Columbia Gas, I worked as a laborer before being promoted to plant supervisor. I used to hold workplace safety meetings once a month, but then the Parkinson's symptoms began to affect my self-esteem. I just didn't have the confidence to get up in front of the men anymore to give the talks. I was starting to shake more, and the tremor in my left hand was increasing, which was making my writing worse, too. Just after 1990, I concluded that I couldn't work anymore and I made plans to retire. I was exactly 55 years old when I officially retired.

After I stopped working, I experienced a bit of depression. I got through it because of my faith, which helped me a lot, and also my wife. She would always remind me that it wasn't as bad as it seemed. She helped me to keep my perspective. For instance, if I was holding up the line in a store my wife would say, "Don't worry about it, take your time, they'll wait." It takes one good brain—that is my wife's—to help me get over most of my hurdles.

I got involved with a clinical study at the University of West Virginia that was also being done in more than 50 other universities. There were 25 participants at each university. The study was to examine Apomorphine, which is a 'rescue' drug used in England that helps when other drugs get less effective over time. The study started in 2003, and it ended up lasting for 40 months.

Dr. Ludwig Gutmann, who coordinated the study, invited me to one of his university classes to demonstrate to students how quickly the apomorphine worked on me. My wife took me there—I had to use a wheelchair to get into the classroom. Dr. Gutmann told the students all about Apomorphine. Then my wife put the needle into my arm and gave me a shot. In about five minutes I got out of the wheelchair and walked effortlessly in front of the class. I felt like a college professor for a moment.

The study is now completed and the drugs are FDA-approved so I still use them. I can tell when my medicine is wearing off and it is at that time that I take a shot. The needle is very small—like an insulin needle. Either I give myself the needle or my wife injects me—I get about two hours of energy out of it. It takes effect in about three minutes, and then I can do whatever I was doing before. Yesterday I cut my lawn for an hour and a half and then I started to feel my medicine wearing off, so I took another shot and I was OK to finish.

The Apomorphine has just made my life so much easier. I prefer using a needle regularly versus having surgery. I still take a lot of medicine on top of the Apomorphine. It takes a total of thirteen pills just to get me started in the morning.

Another thing that I believe has helped me a lot is a special fruit juice that one of the girls at our church introduced me to. I take two ounces three times a day and I have been drinking it for about a year with no side effects. It works for me because it gives me energy and makes me feel like I want to do things.

I have never wanted to blame anybody for my situation and I don't have time to look to others for inspiration. I just keep busy. I'm not one to sit around and watch television. I like to travel. This year I've been to Canada for a week, Aruba in the summer, and Mexico in the fall. I also visited a town called Tillman Island on Chesapeake Bay where, for 16 years, I have attended an annual event with about 20 friends where we fish, eat and have a few drinks.

I have fished since I was a boy. I still love to fish—mainly for trout—but these days, it just takes a little longer for me to get ready. I like getting up early and catching the fish, fixing our own shore lunch, and cooking what we catch. Deer hunting is a favorite activity of mine, too. I happily get up at five o'clock in the morning to go hunting and I have no trouble staying in a tree stand until early afternoon. I take my medication every two hours, although it can be a bit of a challenge getting it out of my pocket without moving too much.

You need to find things to laugh at. For 46 years, my wife has made me laugh about something at least once a day. I have had great support from my kids and family. We have four children and three grandchildren. My two daughters keep a close eye on me and they are always asking me, "Why didn't you call?" or telling me, "You shouldn't go there." They should have been FBI agents.

I am the cook of the family. When I go down to see my doctor I usually take him something to eat, like pepperoni rolls or other homemade things. Stuffed grape leaves are one of my specialties—you haven't lived until you've eaten them. Middle Eastern food is what I like to cook. I learned to cook when my mother broke her collarbone. We had always had homemade bread to eat up to that point and then suddenly we didn't have bread for a couple of months. One night my mother said to me, "Why don't you come up tonight and I will teach you how to make bread." That was about 40 years ago, and I have been baking ever since.

On the negative side, the thing that gets me down the most is all the money spent on research in so many places—not just Parkinson's—and yet it seems we have not had a major cure since polio. Advances have been made in many areas, but it seems there is never a complete cure. It is important to be realistic that a cure for Parkinson's may be more than five years away. I have seen a lot of 'five years' go by already. Sometimes I get a little worried or depressed wondering about what is down the road for me, but I try not to think about it too often. That being said, I think it is important to look on the bright side—maybe they will find something in the near future.

After I was diagnosed, I found a local Parkinson's support group and I decided to attend some of their meetings. Through the group, I have learned a lot of things about Parkinson's. The first coordinator we had always started the meetings with a joke or two. When you get 30 or 40 people laughing, it just feels good.

It is important to take care of yourself. I go every Thursday for exercise classes at the Presbyterian Home of Washington. It is close to two hours of exercise, and it helps a lot. If you take your medication properly, exercise, and watch your diet, you can go on without too many problems.

John Thomas is enjoying his retirement, and he is looking forward to continuing to travel, hunt, fish, and spend time with his family and grandchildren.

CHAPTER FIFTEEN

LINDA COOPER

"Your history doesn't have to be your destiny."

Linda Cooper was diagnosed with Parkinson's disease in 2002. She is 50 years old.

A typical work day for me was getting up at 4:30 in the morning, exercising for one hour and then arriving at work between 6:30 and 7:00 a.m. I was the Executive Director of The Progress Center in Longview, Washington. It is a center for developmentally-delayed newborns, infants and toddlers with disabilities that helps both children and their families. The organization had 17 different sources of funding, so there was always a multitude of reports and monitoring summaries due. I would do a lot of the report writing before the bulk of the staff arrived at 8:30 a.m. I also managed relationships with line supervisors and employees. Around 3 p.m., I would take a break when the Center went out and then I would come back at 5:30 and button things up for an hour. I was very happy to have had the opportunity to work there serving the children and families as well as the employees.

In the late 90s, I experienced depression and had many little symptoms, such as being unable to swing my arm, losing my sense of smell, and being unable to focus or multi-task as well as I used to. However, I was consumed with raising my kids, working and trying to keep a mediocre marriage together, so I just let things pass. But then I started to notice a tremor and pain in my hips and legs. I couldn't deny that something was going on. I did some research—like lots of us 'Parkies' tend to do—and I could read the writing on the wall. I was officially diagnosed with Parkinson's disease in August of 2002. I should have known this would be the outcome—my mother, brother, grandmother, and aunt all had Parkinson's.

On April 22, 2005, my mother died—suffering from the same disease that I had. In my mother's final evening, I lay in bed with her and hugged her. I told her what a wonderful mom she was and how I was going to be fine and that she had lots of people who needed her on the other side. I held her until she died. I wrote a journal entry that night:

4-22-05

I sit in the quiet of the hospice room, my mother dying of the disease that is also robbing me of my independence, clarity of thought and physical abilities. To see her struggle with every breath, muscles paralyzed while her limbs shake uncontrollably seems too cruel a way to die.

I look into the very first set of eyes that met me as I entered this world. The very eyes that have never made me feel a failure or shame but have only encouraged me and loved me. The very same eyes that have seen both her sons laid to rest.

I am planning to donate her brain to the study of Parkinson's disease. To discuss the details at this time seems cruel and morbid. Yet we both would stop at nothing to find the cure to this insidious curse. I touch her head and hope that science appreciates the gift that she is giving them.

My blessing is she has never known of my diagnosis. I could spare her that.

My husband and I lived on the border of Oregon and Washington in a town called Clatskanie with a population of 1,500 people. At one point, I was also on the city council there and I helped on a number of public boards. My first husband was a very kind person and I could not have found a better father for our three children. We started having a bumpy time in our marriage in the early 90s. We pulled it together for a bit but then things went downhill after I was diagnosed with Parkinson's. We divorced after 27 years of marriage.

After being diagnosed, I had a lot of pain, especially in my legs and hip, and it turned out that I also had cognitive impairment and significant short-term impairment. I resigned from my job and applied for disability in May 2005. I was sent to an independent doctor and had to undergo six hours of neuropsychological testing because my Parkinson's displayed itself in non-motor symptoms, making it difficult for Social Security to measure and understand my symptoms. Social Security case managers also talked to people at my work. It took a while but I was finally approved for disability in January 2006.

I used to like walking long distances. Before Parkinson's, I enjoyed meeting a girlfriend and going walking and talking for two hours—not going to happen now. I liked to go to the theater to watch a show. Now when I try to attend, either I fall asleep or it feels like I have 'ants in my legs' and I can't sit still.

I have made a decision that the glass is going to be half-full and that I will make the best out of it. It is a conscious effort to do this. And that's not to say that some days I don't just sit down with the biggest gin and tonic you have ever seen and wallow in self-pity. But that doesn't solve the problem.

Your history doesn't have to be your destiny. I have lots of wonderful things to look forward to. Although Parkinson's is part of my life, it is not my whole life. I have three children whom I love dearly—and my new husband, Michael, who also has Parkinson's. He is further along with the disease in some ways but he doesn't have the short-term cognitive issues that I deal with. He has more significant motor issues and on and off times. So actually it works out really well being together because if I can't remember, he can. I've been given a gift that is beyond compare in Michael. I am very thankful for that.

We both go to the gym every day and do about a half-hour of cardio on whichever machine we happen to step on, followed by free weights and then yoga or Pilates. So basically, we do the triad of cardio, stretching, and strength work. I used to exercise for cosmetic reasons. I still care what I look like, but now it's far more than cosmetic—it's therapeutic and it's a necessity.

Michael and I recently moved to Southern California and are going to be doing quite a bit of work with the Orange County National Parkinson Foundation, helping support groups. There's nothing better than getting outside of yourself and doing something to assist other people. What I can do now is use the skills that I was once paid for to help others. Like they say, volunteerism is the price you pay for taking up space on this earth.

Parkinson's is known as the silent magician. When people get to a point of having tremors or discomfort they tend to drop out of sight. Unless you are at a Parkinson's convention, you don't see too many people with Parkinson's out in public. It's not like cancer where patients wear their baldness proudly. It is important for Parkinson's patients to be out in public every day and to be ambassadors for our cause.

People with Parkinson's need to create their own care plan and team, and they need to be in charge of it. Don't be afraid to seek alternative healthcare like acupuncture, massage or naturopaths. There are a lot of different ways to treat Parkinson's. I believe that you shouldn't take medication until you really have to. It is your life and your body—you need to be in control of that and not let someone else lead you by the hand. There are people who can assist you along the way, but the key is that you stay in charge and use all the 'consultants and advisors' that are at your disposal.

In my life, I never planned to take this journey. It's kind of like a well-known analogy that states: I planned to go to California, but instead I ended up in Holland where the language is different, the people are different but nice and caring, and the food tastes different—but good. Maybe someday I will go back to California but for now I am in Holland, and I'm adjusting to Holland okay.

Linda Cooper married Michael O'Leary on September 22, 2006. Along with her new husband, she continues to be active in lobbying both state and federal governments and she has also spoken at Parkinson's young-onset conferences throughout the country.

CHAPTER SIXTEEN

DR. DAVID HEYDRICK

"I think I have what you have."

Dr. David Heydrick was diagnosed with Parkinson's disease in 2003. He is 44 years old.

I love baseball. While in college, I pitched competitively— I was known more for my accuracy than the speed of my pitches. Being a baseball pitcher helped me to develop the ability to focus when under pressure, and it also taught me invaluable lessons about how to work as part of a team.

In 1987, I completed a Master's degree in Mechanical Engineering and went to work for the Department of Defense. One night in the fall of 1992, I couldn't sleep, so I was sitting on the steps outside my townhouse, contemplating life—my wife calls it my "early mid-life crisis"—when it became clear to me that I should be doing more to help people. I decided to apply to medical school. I was one of those people who applied with the stereotypical line saying, "I want to be a doctor so that I can help people"—but I really meant it. I applied, and was accepted, to the University of Maryland. After nine years of medical school, internship, neurology residency and neuromuscular fellowship, I was officially a neurologist in June 2002.

I immediately started working in a private practice. One month later, I was driving home after work and I was testing myself by doing finger-tapping. I was slow on my right side and that concerned me because I had been a right-handed pitcher so, if anything, that should have been my fast side. I put that concern to the back of my mind for the next few months. However, in January 2003, a right arm tremor showed up. Food was dropping from my fork before it reached my mouth. I did my best to deny the existence and significance of the tremor.

I was working as a general neurologist, and our practice saw a variety of patients. I had about ten Parkinson's patients at that time, plus I had seen quite a few through my residency. I distinctly remember a very pleasant elderly patient who came in to the practice every four to six months. Her Parkinson's was progressing, but she was always upbeat. She came in for an appointment and, as she sat in her chair and I sat in mine, I noticed that our hand tremors were almost totally in synch. With her sitting in front of me, it was like looking in the mirror. I said to her, "I think I have what you have." I asked her, "Is there any way that you can stop your tremor?" She answered, "Yes," and moved her hand to show me how she did it. I tried the same thing, and my tremor stopped temporarily. It was a simple but defining moment.

My colleagues thought that I had Parkinson's and I now suspected that I did, too. I was familiar with Parkinson's because my grandfather had it. However, it took an F-dopa

PET scan to convince me that I did indeed have it. I was officially diagnosed October 10, 2003.

After being diagnosed, symptoms progressed quickly and started encompassing my entire right side. The leg tremor became worse and, within six months, I had developed a horrendous facial tremor that was very debilitating. The symptoms were making it extremely difficult to write and, for a short time, it was impossible for me to drive or give speeches. I also had restless and fractured sleep during that time, so there was a fatigue element, too.

I was on track to becoming a full partner in the private practice by July 2005. But, in the spring of 2004, it became obvious that I could not keep up with my expected workload. My fellow doctors at the practice and I agreed that we should part ways. I bullheadedly decided to start my own practice, working as a solo practitioner. I did that for six months and, although the practice worked out from a patient-interaction side, it was too stressful for me and I experienced depression. Around autumn 2004, I declined precipitously. The right-sided tremor was out of control and the medicine was not working. Physically and emotionally, it was all I could do to get out of bed.

I felt that the only way I could fight back against the fatigue and the pain was to diminish my motor symptoms—so I decided to get Deep Brain Stimulation (DBS) surgery. I concluded that it was a good option because I was tremor-predominant and young. My fears of the surgery were quickly stamped out when I calculated the risk was far outweighed by the potential benefit. I had the surgery at the Cleveland Clinic Foundation on January 19, 2005.

One month later, I went back to Cleveland and had the

device programmed. I was lying on the table in the exam room and the tremors were actively 'doing their thing'—and then the programmer found the right settings and all of a sudden the tremors stopped. It was amazing and I was exhilarated. The day before, I had come to Cleveland with a debilitating tremor and I returned to Baltimore the following day on a plane, sitting very quietly and calmly. This was a whole new experience for me because I had lived with tremors every waking hour for the last two years. It felt fantastic to once again be able to play baseball with my sons Scott and Christopher.

Eventually, the tremor progressed to my left side, so I had a second DBS operation in September 2005. It was also a success. After my recovery from the DBS surgery, I was able to go back to work roughly six to eight hours a week as a neurologist. I also began developing an exercise and nutrition program for my own health preservation.

I was asked to be part of the first-ever World Parkinson Congress, which happened in February 2006 in Washington D.C. They wanted me to talk, as both a patient and a doctor, about being proactive regarding Parkinson's. I had spent the year accumulating a framework of scientifically-based studies that I put together as the best ways to battle Parkinson's. I was lying in bed one night a few weeks prior to the speech, feeling that I needed a concept that tied all of my speaking points together. Somehow the food pyramid popped into my mind—it was a 'eureka moment'—for that was the birth of the concept that I discuss in my speeches, The Parkinson's Pyramid™.

The Parkinson's Pyramid™ is simply connecting the dots between the pieces of scientific knowledge that are out in the public domain. It is comprised of several elements, namely focused nutrition, varieties of exercise, stress management, and specific symptom management. In my speeches, I try to get across that The Parkinson's Pyramid™ is a package deal. It is integrated medicine or, more simply, a rational lifestyle approach.

My philosophy on medication—and there is some physiology behind this—is that you should try to be on the lowest effective dose. I actually take no Parkinson's medication. How do you do this? For starters, I have come to believe passionately in the importance of stress management. Exercise is also critical—aerobic exercise can decrease the amount of medicine you have to take. In the winter, I am active six to seven days per week. My schedule varies from cycling on a stationary bike or running on a treadmill in my basement, to using machines at the gym. I wear a heart rate monitor and I do a half-hour to one hour per day. Twice a week I try to do high-intensity weightlifting. I also do plenty of stretching and take Tai Chi classes. My nutritional plan is centered on anti-oxidant and anti-inflammatory foods. You have to attack Parkinson's from many directions.

I believe that, from the day of diagnosis, we should be proactive about our health. There are 8,760 hours in a year and appointments with the neurologist only account for about 4 hours. Therefore, for the remaining 8,756 hours we have to take responsibility for our health.

My health improved so much that in the summer of 2006, my oldest son Scott and I were in Iowa cycling 450 miles across the state to raise money for Parkinson's. One day, we had finished our daily 70-mile ride, and Scott and I were completely exhausted as we pressed on to get to the host family's house. We thought it was very close—just over one hill—and that we would be able to spot the house by the big white support trailer that would be parked out front. We were mistaken—we cycled over hill after hill, all the while gradually cycling uphill. Physically, we were drained and down to our last bits of energy. Psychologically, we were discouraged because we would bike over a hill and think that we saw the trailer, but then our hopes would be dashed when it turned out that it was simply a road sign or something else. We went over thirteen hills and each time we were disappointed. Finally, we spotted the house and, as we arrived, we raised our arms in victory as if we had won the Tour de France. We charged down the hill to the driveway and collapsed on the ground, exhausted but jubilant that we had finally arrived.

Living with Parkinson's is very similar to that cycling experience. It is often a difficult uphill ride. We experience many disappointments but we keep going. We receive reports from the media that a cure is near, yet it seems that we are constantly being disappointed. Ultimately, we keep going—and I am sure that eventually our persistence will be rewarded and that we will raise our arms in victory!

I hope that the knowledge that I have accumulated will help others by 'flattening out the hills' along the way and making the 'ride' easier.

Dr. David Heydrick is currently writing a book called **Back in the Game: The Parkinson's Pyramid™**, *and he continues to deliver speeches across the country. He was the keynote speaker at the Muhammad Ali Parkinson's Center educational symposium, which took place in February 2007.*

CHAPTER SEVENTEEN

PATTY MEEHAN

"Don't go through it alone."

Patty Meehan was diagnosed with Parkinson's disease in 2005. She is 50 years old.

I started out working as a teller and gradually moved up, going from bank to bank. However, my true passion was plants and flowers so I left the banking world. I eventually ended up working at one of Michigan's biggest nurseries where I became an Advanced Master Gardener in 1999. It was fun working there—I loved the freedom of being outside.

The owner of the plant nursery would sometimes have me work on his personal garden. They had two llamas to protect their sheep from coyotes. I would go there and I'd spend more time with the llamas than I would completing my gardening chores. In 2001, my husband and I moved out to the country and bought a 100-year-old farmhouse with a barn in the back. I felt that we had to get something to fill the barn so we purchased Moondance, Flash, Xipe and Treacle—four llamas.

I help out at a nursing home and one time for 'pet therapy' I wanted to bring a unique animal—not a dog or a cat. So my husband and I decided to take a couple of our llamas. It was such a thrill to see the people smile the minute they saw them. The llamas are like a cross between a very big cat and a teddy bear—calm, curious, gentle and very loving. And in my opinion, extremely cute, too!

My symptoms started in the fall of 2004. I first noticed that my left arm wasn't swinging when I walked. I would try to wave at the llamas with my left hand but my hand would just stay there—like I was giving somebody a high-five. I decided to see a neurologist but I didn't like the first one I saw because, twenty minutes into my initial visit, he told me to come back in three months. I found another neurologist and he spent nearly two hours with me before giving me the diagnosis that I indeed had Parkinson's disease.

I already knew a great deal about Parkinson's because my mother had been diagnosed with Parkinson's in 1973 at the age of 49. She lived with it for 28 years before passing away in 2001—approximately ten years after my father had passed away with Alzheimer's.

I hit the wall upon hearing that I had Parkinson's and was pretty down and out initially because I remembered all that my mom went through. I thought, "How can I put my husband and brother through this again—after they had been through it with my mother." I keep thinking back to the time my mom was diagnosed, when I was in high school. She fought depression and would get up during the night, not being able to sleep, and just sit at the dining room table and cry. I knew she was afraid—I am, too.

Fairly quickly, I decided to keep reminding myself that I have Parkinson's and that Parkinson's doesn't have me. I will deal with it. I can't get it out of me or throw it away so I just have to live my life the best I can. It's not going to get me down. I have my moments where I feel sorry for myself but I tell myself to snap out of it.

My husband is nine years younger than me—we married in August 1995, ten years before I was diagnosed. I love having an early morning coffee with him while we enjoy our little piece of property. He makes me laugh and keeps me going when I am slowing down. He knows what my mom went through and lets me try everything first and helps me only if I ask for his assistance. My older brother is also there for me anytime, which is a very comforting feeling. I have a strong faith—I feel that I am on this path in life for a reason.

Handwriting is a challenge—I used to write letters all the time, but now I type them. Sometimes typing is even hard, because I will mistakenly put my baby finger on the 'a' and it will go all across the page aaaaaaaaaaaaaaaaaaa. Initially, when my tremors were really bad I would sit on my hand or put it in my pocket. I was embarrassed to go anywhere because of the tremors. Most of my friends know that I have it now and they are very supportive.

I was always multitasking. I now tell myself, "Okay Patty, do one thing at a time, you'll get there, just do one thing at a time." I was so used to quickly doing many domestic things like cleaning the house, doing the laundry and mowing the grass, but I have now accepted that I can't do that as fast anymore. I am slowly learning patience.

Exercise is a great way to fight back at Parkinson's. I get on the treadmill each day and walk three to five miles. I force myself to do this. It is a discipline thing—I have to do it. I don't feel as stiff and I think that my gait has improved.

Communicating can be kind of hard at times. We were running around the other morning and we stopped at a Dairy Queen. I wanted a Pumpkin Pie Blizzard and I couldn't get the word Pumpkin out. I went pump-pump-pump-pump-pump. It is frustrating when you want to say something but the words just don't come out right.

I now do quite a bit of volunteer work. I visit a local nursing home every Thursday to do a little bit of horticultural therapy with the residents. It is so rewarding to see them smile and laugh at some of the projects we do. During the growing season, I tend to their courtyard garden. I also deliver Meals on Wheels around here. It is such a joy to see and help people who are shut in and who can't get out. They always want to sit and talk with you. It gives you a great feeling knowing you are helping someone.

I made a conscious choice that I am going to live a full life with Parkinson's and that I will not let it become an excuse. I used to spend eight hours in the garden—now I spend only three before I get tired or sore. I also do ceramics, which is a challenge with the tremors but I keep doing it and now instead of doing tiny paintings, I do large jobs which are easier. I am not going to stop doing ceramics or gardening. Don't sit around—follow your passion and don't quit because you have Parkinson's.

Learn everything that you can about Parkinson's. I recommend getting into a support group because they are like another family and all the people in it understand what you're going through. My mom used to always say, "I feel so shaky today," and I'd look at her and say, "Mom, you're not even shaking." She would insist she was shaking inside. Other people with Parkinson's would have better understood and empathized with what she was telling me. I now know what she was talking about because sometimes I get like that where I feel a terrible shaking inside—like I am in a blender or something—although outwardly nothing shows.

Regardless of whether you decide to get involved with a support group, I think it is important to have a friend, a doctor or a psychiatrist you can talk to. Also communicate to your family about what you are going through—just don't go through it alone.

Patty Meehan stays active by helping out with various charities and support groups. Her llamas are now regular visitors to the nursing home.

CHAPTER EIGHTEEN

NICK KAETHLER

"I was not beating as many kids at ping-pong and my singing voice was slipping a bit."

Nick Kaethler was diagnosed with Parkinson's disease in 1998. He is 66 years old.

I was born on May 8, 1940 in the Dnieper area of Ukraine to German parents. The Second World War came to our part of the country the same year. When the Germans were coming, the Russians took anyone of German descent who was living in Ukraine and put them on a train to Siberia—60 of our family members were sent there. Most died in the next few years.

My father ended up being imprisoned and sentenced to 25 years in jail by the Russians while my mother escaped the Russians by traveling from Russia to Germany on horse-drawn carriages or trains. She was a 25-year-old refugee who had my two kid brothers plus her cousin's two children, who were five and three years old and she was pregnant. She gave birth to a daughter on the way to Germany but tragically the baby froze to death. I ended up in the best German children's hospital suffering from tuberculosis. Later we were all put into an orphanage and stayed there for two years while my mother received treatment on her face, which had frozen during the arduous journey to Germany. Parkinson's is nothing compared to those experiences.

We emigrated from Germany to Canada in 1948, but just before we left we found out that my father was still alive in a Russian prison. In 1956, Khrushchev came into power and there was a glasnost-like time where he cut all political sentences in half. My father was released at that time but, because it was during the Cold War, it was very difficult to get out of Russia. He was not of much use to the Russians economically as he had tuberculosis, which is probably why they finally let him out of the country in 1965.

My father finally arrived in Toronto and was fed Kentucky Fried Chicken for his first Canadian meal. It was quite a surprise when he showed up at our door in Kitchener-Waterloo. Fortunately, my mother had not remarried. Her statement on the timing of his arrival to Canada—when my brothers and I were in our twenties—was, "God must have known what He was doing. I don't know how I could have raised three teenage boys and retrained one husband at the same time."

In the 60s I sang professionally in Toronto, spending four years with the Elmer Iseler Festival Singers. I moved to Guelph in 1969 and met my current wife, June, in 1973 in the university choir—I pulled her hat over her eyes and she pulled the wool over my eyes. Over the years, I directed choirs and taught at high schools and universities before becoming the music director for 60 schools in the district.

My Parkinson's symptoms started to show in 1997. At the time, I was the Lieutenant Governor for Kiwanis and I was required to give speeches, which I used to enjoy making. However, I became paranoid and I felt that my speeches were becoming incoherent and ineffective. Several other things confirmed to me that there was a problem. Waking up in the middle of the night and not being able to turn over was not normal for a healthy person. I started to be afraid to do things in public and I was shuffling when I walked. Also, my singing voice started to lose its power. I lost confidence, energy, and intensity.

My general practitioner at first told me that I was just getting old. Eventually, he referred me to a neurologist, who recognized Parkinson's disease and prescribed Levodopa. I took my three pills per day and magically felt better. I didn't know much about Parkinson's. It was a bit of a relief to learn what was causing my symptoms because I finally had a name for what was happening to me. I could now be a bit more proactive about how I was going to live with it.

June and I were worried about the risk of my health declining swiftly even though I was doing fine, so we sold everything and bought a motor home. For four years we traveled and saw virtually every state and province. I had been a ping-pong champion at university and after being diagnosed with Parkinson's, ping-pong became a barometer to indicate how well I was doing physically. I figured I was doing OK when I won a Silver medal in ping-pong at the Senior Winter Olympics in Brownsville, Texas.

We felt that I was strong enough to go somewhere to teach. I tested myself by supply teaching for eleven weeks and it showed me that I still had the energy. We applied to teach English as a Second Language *(ESL)* in Korea but they wouldn't have us because we were too old. When the placement person for Korea found out I was 62 years old, he laughed out loud and said, "We put people on the shelf at that age." I said, "Not me." We applied to forty other places that wanted ESL teachers. I was finally accepted through a Mennonite agency, the China Educational Exchange.

In February 2003 we went to a Sichuan teaching university—it had 70,000 students by the time we left. It was a province in the center of China and the capital city was Chengdu which is a 'small' big city of over ten million people. Communicating was not too much of a problem because the students came to university with six years of English. There were a few other teachers that helped us get oriented. We enjoyed ourselves very much and suffered little culture shock.

During the two and a half years in China, my meds did not change but my symptoms did. On annual visits to Canada I would get a year's supply of meds and the doctor said I was the same but I really wasn't—I was going downhill. I needed more sleep. I was not beating as many kids at ping-pong and my singing voice was slipping a bit.

When I came home in September 2005, I was having difficulty finding the right words when I spoke. People all thought I looked pale—I was not 'with it'. One time I fell asleep while eating dinner and visiting people. I realized I was not in as good a shape as I should be, so I went to a doctor and had my first-ever thorough checkup to establish my health baseline and it helped a lot.

Occasionally, I still cannot find the right words. I get frustrated sometimes at my lack of ability to multitask. I have become very single-minded. What I did automatically before, I can now still do but I have to consciously think about what I am doing. It is like switching from an automatic car to using a gearshift—and not just a simple gearshift but one that has 18 gears. Trying to handle all the shifts is tiring.

Whatever you do, get the right medicine. Get help from a doctor who is a specialist in the area of Parkinson's. I feel that I have markedly improved over the last year because of different meds, voice therapy, and maybe even because the air is cleaner in Canada than in China. A positive attitude and a strong faith have also helped me tremendously.

You can't change the state that you are in but you can change your response to that state. You can control and do things that will make you more cheerful. I believe you become more cheerful when you are helping others because you are not thinking about yourself.

It is important to stay both mentally and physically active and don't ever lose your sense of humor. Believe in yourself.

Over the years, Nick Kaethler has won awards for his singing, and today, despite his voice not being as powerful, he still loves to sing classical music. His current favorite song is, **To Dream The Impossible Dream.**

Nick and June Kaethler currently run the Parkinson's Support Group for Guelph & Wellington, Ontario.

CHAPTER NINETEEN

TOM O'DONNELL

"If you were 35 years or older, I would swear that you have Parkinson's disease."

Tom O'Donnell was diagnosed with Parkinson's disease in 1991. He is 44 years old.

I attended Buffalo State College and played football but, after one year, I left college and joined the army in 1982. I became a military policeman working out of Fort Jackson, South Carolina. While I was there, I would shake a bit, especially when I was doing things like tearing down an M16 rifle for speed. One time, I was investigating a burglary at the main PX *(Post Exchange)* on our base. As I went to investigate, my knees started to shake like Bugs Bunny in a cartoon. I never worried about the shaking because I was only in my early 20s.

I got married to my high school sweetheart Katie in 1984 and, one year later, I left the army and went to work as a car salesman. I sold everything from Toyotas to Dodges. I had been earning $13,000 a year in the army and then all of a sudden I was making $27,000 a year. I felt like the richest guy on earth!

Fast forward to 1988. Katie and I were doing very well as a double-income, no-kids couple. We had new cars, nice clothes and we were having lots of fun. In April of that year, I was bringing a cup of coffee to a customer and I noticed that my left hand was shaking. I thought it was no big deal, and that it probably was because I had been lifting weights a little earlier that day. When you are 26 years old and your arm shakes, you just put your hand in your pocket and don't worry about it.

Around that time, an acquaintance who was a neurologist told me I should see someone about my shaking. I blew him off—I didn't see any reason to see a doctor about it. Then, two months later, I noticed that I was scuffing my left foot on the ground, like some kids do. So, with no real concern at all, I decided to get it checked out. They gave me a CAT scan, thinking that I might have Multiple Sclerosis—mainly because Buffalo had a Multiple Sclerosis rate that was double the national average. Another theory was that I could have ruptured a disc in my neck or that I had a tumor on my brain. The MRIs came back negative. The doctor said, "If you were 35 years or older, I would swear that you have Parkinson's disease."

I got accepted for a job working in the prisons for the New York State correctional office and on December 10, 1989, I went to work at the only women's maximum correctional facility in New York State. It was a nightmare. Those women fought at the drop of a hat and were very dangerous. I worked there for three months, nineteen days and seven hours.

My next place of work was Mohawk Correctional Facility, which housed men. I thought the guys would be worse, but I was totally wrong. They fought a lot less and mainly kept to themselves. Over the next two years, my symptoms got worse—both my arms were shaking badly. Luckily, I had a way of hiding my shakes from the inmates by keeping my arms behind me. It wasn't until 1991 that I was officially diagnosed with Parkinson's.

I stayed at Mohawk until I went on sick leave in the spring of 1993. During my time on sick leave, I fished for trout with my neighbor for 72 days straight. My neighbor had to put the minnows and worms on the hook—I was squirming and shaking as much as the worms were.

Earlier that year I had gone to a symposium and listened to a man speaking there who had such bad dyskinesia that I thought he would fall off the stage. I shook hands with him and I gave him my number. He called me a year later and said he had undergone stereotactic surgery. I went to see him and he seemed like a new man. He looked so calm, he could have split a diamond. I decided then that I would get stereotactic brain surgery, too.

Before I left work, the correctional officers got together and pooled the vacation time they had accumulated, and they donated it to me to help me afford to go out west and have the surgery done. I traveled with my dad, my sister-in-law and my wife. My dad was not as confident about the procedure—unbeknownst to me, he had actually planned with an undertaker on how to get a casket back from California!

During the surgery they went too far into my brain and nipped my optic nerve. That resulted in me temporarily losing my peripheral vision, although it has come back over time. I still have some spasms that force my eyes to close, though. During the operation, I also had a surgically-induced stroke on my left side. It was a nightmare day. As a result of the operation, there would be times when I would be walking in a parking lot and bump into the mirrors of parked cars because I had lost all feeling and peripheral vision.

When I got home, I was not sure what I could do. My left side was semi-paralyzed. I thought that maybe I could help coach football, and so I went back to my old high school, Lancaster High School, as an assistant wide receiver coach. It was great to be with the kids. Afterwards, I created a scholarship called the Coaches' Choice Award. Each year, I donate $1,000 and the coaches select a deserving kid and give them the award and the money.

Despite the problems that resulted from my first operation, I went back six months later for a second operation. My doctor told me not to go. She said it was too big a risk but, in my mind, there was no other alternative. I had to have the operation simply because I could not look after my wife and kids if I did not have a job. On February 2, 1994, I went back into surgery. This time another doctor did the operation and it worked out well. The shaking on my right side lessened.

I eventually resumed working at Mohawk and worked there until 1998, at which point I resigned. I told my deputy superintendent, "I am starting to get dizzy, and it's not safe for me to work anymore. It's time." Unfortunately, I only had nine years of work experience and I needed ten years for benefits. The union held a fundraiser for me, and they raised $14,000. They told me they had walked around the jail and people had donated time one day here, two weeks there—enough time to add one year to my nine years of experience so that I would have the ten years necessary to qualify for benefits. I asked them, "Why me?" And they answered, "Because you never complained."

Katie and I have two kids, a 14-year-old daughter and a 10-year-old son. Of the 22 years we have been married, I have had Parkinson's for 18 of them. My goals are to continue to take care of my family, and to dance with my daughter at her wedding. Hopefully she won't get married until she is 35.

I look at it this way. I have a disease that is very hard to explain. If I were to tell people how I actually feel, people might be very depressed. At this moment, every inch of my body is doing one thing or another. Why should I tell them that and bring them down? So why not say that I feel great instead? It's a good ice-breaker, because everyone wants to know why I feel so great.

Parkinson's has helped me to take the blinders off. It allowed me to realize that there was more to life than how I was living at the time. My feeling of being immortal has ended. I have been humbled. I now understand that we can break. It made me realize that I was here for another reason—to speak and be a voice for those who cannot communicate because of Parkinson's disease.

If you get depressed, do something. Do whatever it takes to make you feel better. It is easier to handle Parkinson's by doing things and keeping active than by sitting in a chair and being depressed. Never ever give up. Parkinson's may steal your mind and your body—but it will never touch your heart and your soul.

Quitting is the harder way out.

Tom O'Donnell's Coaches' Choice Award is now in its 13th year. Tom O'Donnell is also a charter member of the Central New York Parkinson's Support Group, and he is a co-founder of the Parkinson's Association of Western New York.

CHAPTER TWENTY

CHERIE ZAUN

"You're nuts. I'm an athlete. I don't have Parkinson's!"

Cherie Zaun was diagnosed with Parkinson's disease in 2003. She is 55 years old.

My older brother Rick and I played little league baseball when we were kids. Although I was better than he was, league officials decided it was too dangerous for a girl to play baseball and so I had to quit. Rick *(Dempsey)* got to continue on in baseball and later became a famous catcher, playing for over 20 years in the major leagues with teams like the New York Yankees and the Baltimore Orioles.

I was a volleyball player all through school. In those days, women didn't have professional volleyball teams or else I might have done that. I didn't take up golf until I was 21 years old. I lived next door to a golf course, so I thought I might as well give the sport a try. I went over with my children in a stroller and started hitting golf balls. A pro came out and said, "You're pretty good at that, you should do something with it. You can make a lot of money with your playing ability." Bingo! I spent the next year hitting golf balls and then turned pro at the end of the year. I qualified for a couple of Ladies Professional Golf Association *(LPGA)* tournaments and then later I went on to play in other tournaments.

When I was trying to play professionally, there were very few other golfers who had children. It was difficult to get out there and play a lot while also being a mother because there wasn't child care at the courses. I got a lot of babysitters and I took the kids most places with me when they were little. They would sit and watch me hit golf balls. I ended up retiring in 1980, when my kids were getting to the age where they would be in school. My old coach from the Bel-Air Country Club, Eddie Merrins, jokingly told me to come back when my children were fully grown. Sixteen years later, I showed up at the course ready to go back to work. Eddie took one look at me and said, "I am not surprised to see you back!"

In 1996, at the age of 44, I officially resumed my golf career and competed in Futures Tour events. When I came back to golf, I would play and I would be fine, but then all of a sudden I would just hit a funky, crazy shot. I lost some feeling in my right hand but the sensation was very slight and I wasn't aware of why it was happening at the time. Sometimes I would just have problems feeling comfortable with the club in my hand. Looking back, these were probably early indications of Parkinson's.

I was playing in a tournament in Ohio when, after I hit my tee shot, I walked off the tee block, slipped on the grass and jammed my right side. My shoulder and elbow were very sore but I continued to play. I started holding my right arm up because of the soreness. I went to an orthopedic guy and he gave me some medication that made me feel better. Around the same time, I worked with a physical therapist/trainer and he noticed that I was not moving my right arm anymore. I went to a neurologist in Glendale and he did some tests but couldn't find anything. It didn't get any better so I went to another doctor who examined me and then put me on medication that made me feel nauseous 24 hours a day.

At one tournament, I ended up playing with a pharmacist in a Monday Pro-Am and he asked me, "What are you taking?" because he had noticed I was sick. I told him and he replied, "That's Parkinson's medicine. Do you have Parkinson's?" That was the first I had heard about Parkinson's.

I went back to the doctor who had prescribed the medicine and I asked him if he thought I had Parkinson's. He looked at the wall for probably a good minute before he turned around and said, "Yes, I think you have Parkinson's." I said, "You're nuts. I'm an athlete. I don't have Parkinson's!" I was in complete denial. Six months later, I went to see Dr. Mark Lew, and within five minutes he diagnosed me with Parkinson's just by the way I was moving.

My son was in spring training with the Houston Astros down in Florida. I called him and I said, "Gregg, ask the team doctors if I could be incorrectly diagnosed with Parkinson's disease if I had a pinched nerve." The doctors said yes, most definitely, the diagnosis could be incorrect. When the Astros broke up their spring training camp, I went to Houston and was put through the paces of all the X-rays, and at one point I actually had some hope that the initial diagnosis was wrong. Instead, I soon received confirmation from them that I had Parkinson's. I finally had to accept the diagnosis.

I still compete and play in tournaments, but I have had to change my whole swing to be more left side dominant. I'm currently just trying to figure out how to adjust when I don't feel comfortable on my right side. I could go down to the golf course today and hit some great shots but then I'll set up for a shot and not be able to get the 'feel'. In competition, when the stress kicks in, the right side of my body starts to break down so I try to keep a positive attitude and remind myself that I'm just out having fun.

I'm not going to Q school *(qualifying school for the Futures Tour)* this year because I don't feel comfortable about the progress that I have made with the change in my swing. I won't give up trying, though. I can play well and I can still hit a drive 220 to 230 yards, which is good enough. Golf keeps me going. If I didn't have golf, I would have to find something else athletic to do to fight this disease—it's just in me. I can't give up and quit.

My next-door neighbor had Parkinson's and his wife was in complete denial. She still to this day does not think that he had it but we used to watch him walk up and down the driveway and it seemed pretty obvious that he had Parkinson's. The stigma is with the word 'Parkinson's'. Everybody has to pull a card out of the deck and deal with it in their life and this is mine and that was his. I sometimes have to correct people who say he died of Parkinson's because you don't die of Parkinson's, you die with it. It doesn't kill you, but it sure makes life a challenge.

More and more people are getting diagnosed—by some estimates, every nine minutes a new person is diagnosed with Parkinson's. There are a lot of people with Parkinson's who withdraw because they feel very embarrassed that they have tremors and a lot of other problems. They need to be able to say that they have Parkinson's. We need everyone to understand that it is a real disease and that it is affecting people more and more. We need to create awareness of it so we can find a cure.

I have discovered that I am stronger than I thought I was. I will accept what happens in the future because I don't have a choice. That being said, I will keep trying to play golf and work to raise Parkinson's awareness. I am a mom, a wife, a friend, a daughter, and a sister—all these people in my family count on me to be strong. I'm the one living with Parkinson's and it is something that I have to deal with but I don't want to bring other people down. I want them to be proud of me.

Exercise is so critical to achieving my goals. I want to stay in shape as long as possible so that I can inspire others to fight this disease. My aim is to do whatever I can to create awareness and raise money for research because I believe a cure for Parkinson's would also help lead to a cure for Alzheimer's disease—which is a terrible way to die—and also for Multiple Sclerosis and other diseases.

You can't sit in a recliner and feel sorry for yourself. You have to get out of the chair and live life. Do something about it. You have to keep trying.

In 1976, Cherie Zaun won the Virginia State Open. Now, besides pursuing her golf career as the oldest player on the Futures Tour, Cherie Zaun continues to travel throughout North America, speaking to groups to raise awareness and to help motivate those with Parkinson's.

Her son, Gregg, is a catcher for the Toronto Blue Jays. He has created the Gregg Zaun Foundation that is focused on raising money for Parkinson's research.

CHAPTER TWENTY-ONE

CARROLL NEESEMANN

"Don't quit your job because you are self-conscious about having Parkinson's."

Carroll Neesemann was diagnosed with Parkinson's disease in 1996. He is 66 years old.

For no reason that I can recall other than that my brother had done it before me, I joined the Navy Reserve Officers' Training Corps *(ROTC)* in college. But I soon found that I rather disliked the Navy, which seemed too fancy for me. I switched to the Marine Corps, which suited me far better.

In those days, the military used line officers in lieu of lawyers to represent the troops when they had minor legal issues. I was appointed to represent a few guys who allegedly possessed more than one identity card, and other small cases like that. I enjoyed it immensely, and the experience influenced my decision to attend law school after my time in the service.

Towards the end of my tour of duty in the Marines, I was in Vietnam, based at Chu Lai. One afternoon, I caught a little bit of the shrapnel in my torso from a booby-trapped hand grenade. They did some exploratory abdominal surgery and as a result, I couldn't go back into the field so I was sent home.

Upon returning to Baltimore late in the summer of 1966, I didn't know what to do with myself. I found that I could apply to the University of Maryland School of Law without waiting a year, so I applied and was accepted. I started law school that year. It was not very expensive for me to attend because I was a resident of Maryland. While I was in the Marine Corps my father had died, leaving enough money to take care of our family. My father had left me the cash value of several small insurance policies. That, combined with the GI bill, allowed me to scrape by.

I even had just enough money to buy a cheap flight to Europe during the summer of my second year in law school. I hitchhiked around Europe while waiting for a Marine Corps buddy of mine to join me on the continent. I went to the Spanish island of Majorca and there I met a girl from Finland who was on vacation. She came to the U.S. and visited me a couple of times but then things went chilly for a bit. Luckily for me, we ended up resuming our relationship, and we were married in 1977.

My wife is the love of my life and the best thing that ever happened to me, followed closely by our children. The best part of my life has been raising the kids with my wife. My daughter is now 28 and lives here in Brooklyn, while my son is five years younger and living in Chicago.

In 1996, my Parkinson's symptoms started to appear. I was

driving back to the city from Long Island, holding the steering wheel, when I noticed a tremor in my left hand. I immediately went to my general practitioner, who concluded that I had Parkinson's disease right off the bat— his diagnosis was quickly confirmed by a neurologist. I wasn't overly pleased to hear that I had Parkinson's, although at that time I didn't know that much about it.

Up to that point, I had spent my whole career working in New York City as a litigator—a job that put me under intense pressure. It was typical for me to lie awake in the middle of the night worrying about my cases. Parkinson's made it impossible for me to do that kind of high-stress litigation anymore. However, I had received advice early on—good advice—that a person with Parkinson's disease should—if at all possible—never quit working. I was lucky that I was a partner in a law firm that prided itself on the treatment of its work force. I was also fortunate that over the years I had served from time to time as an arbitrator, so I switched from being a litigator to working as an arbitrator, which was less stressful.

Continuing to work with Parkinson's disease is easier said than done. There is a tendency to feel self-conscious about having Parkinson's, especially if you have a symptom that makes you look 'different', like a tremor, stooped-over posture, a peculiar way of walking or an inability to resume walking after a stop—say, for a traffic light. In the short run, the easy way out is to avoid the embarrassment and quit. But the cost of doing so is high—both from the loss of income and from the impact to one's feelings of self-worth. In any case, I think it is best to continue to do your job as long as you possibly can.

There are practical problems, of course. You may feel sleepy during the day because Parkinson's has kept you up for much of the night. The meds themselves can sometimes contribute to making you feel sleepy. On the other hand, at times you can get a lot of good, productive work done in those wee hours when, at least for me, the symptoms usually leave me alone. And just getting yourself ready to leave the house in the morning is a chore. Shaving can be a challenge, although an electric razor given to me by Santa has helped immensely. There are ways to shortcut some of the preparation process—for example, my shirt takes forever to button, so instead of doing this, I can either wear a shirt without buttons if the job permits or just ask my wife, "Please, button me up."

It is not surprising that many people with Parkinson's choose to hide the fact that they have it as long as possible, or quit work to avoid the complexities of dealing with the issue. I chose to come out of the closet and post my diagnosis in my bio on the Internet. I feel that by doing this, I am implicitly assuring others that I have done my homework to learn about the disease and its effect on me. As well, I am confirming that I still have the ability to do any work that I accept and that I can still function at a high level of competence.

I highly recommend taking time to learn about Parkinson's disease and the ways to combat it. There is a wealth of information—covering symptoms, medications, and also suggestions for coping with the disease on a daily basis— that can be acquired from books, support groups and the Internet.

Shortly after its creation, I became involved with a Parkinson's support group in Brooklyn. The brainchild of our founder and President, Olie Westheimer, is a weekly modern dance class for people with Parkinson's and their caregivers, taught by marvelous dancers from the Mark Morris Dance Group at their facility in Brooklyn. The classes have a certain magical quality that enables persons with Parkinson's to shed their symptoms to a greater or lesser degree and move as they can at no other time during the week. Our support group is comprised of wonderful people who care very much about each other.

The importance of exercise has been universally recognized—recent research seems to indicate that exercise can be neuro-protective and can perhaps slow or stop the progress of the disease. Our support group also has a group exercise program and we are working on developing a more strenuous program to provide aerobics and strength training. It will help anyone who is of middle and older age— especially those with Parkinson's.

Get involved and physical in whatever way you can! Move, walk, dance, exercise. Join something. Don't agonize over 'forgetting' to exercise or missing a meeting. Unfortunately, Parkinson's does not bring with it perfect self-discipline. Just don't quit.

Fight the disease with all your might, but don't be silly about it. Don't waste your time trying to regain the ability to do things perfectly that you simply cannot do well any more—like buttoning your shirt. Try to get over the embarrassment that comes with the Parkinson's territory and contributes to its debilitating effects. For example, when I am speaking to a group of people, I tell them to let me know if I am talking too softly and I will speak up if that is required. There is nothing wrong with acknowledging the facts of Parkinson's and the changes to life that it brings. But try your best to avoid the irresistible temptation to let

Parkinson's be an excuse or a crutch—which is often done by being the first person to bring Parkinson's into a conversation.

Let your objective be more than just becoming the best Parkinson's patient you can be. Try to be the best person you can be—who just happens to have Parkinson's disease.

In the summer of 2006, Carroll Neesemann was listed by New York Magazine as one of the best lawyers in New York for Alternative Dispute Resolution. He continues to practice law as a commercial arbitrator.

CHAPTER TWENTY-TWO

PATRICIA SHERRICK

"I am not going to alter my life and stop doing things that I like to do just because I have Parkinson's."

Patricia Sherrick was diagnosed with Parkinson's disease in 1996. She is 63 years old.

My husband Jim and I married in 1965 and we have five children, who in turn have produced sixteen grandchildren. The biggest challenge during the years we were raising our children was trying to keep food on the table. They are all good kids but, growing up, they kept me very busy. We struggled to make ends meet—at one point I was doing three jobs—but we made it through OK.

In early 1996, I was working in Lima, Ohio in the Smokehouse Meats section of the County Market, where the temperature ranged between 32 to 35 degrees Fahrenheit. It was kept at that temperature because that was where the meat was stored. Most days, I was stuffing meat into casings—my right arm controlling the filling action of the machine and my left arm holding the casings. Doing this put me in an uncomfortable position—I was always leaning to one side. At the end of each day, my body was usually very tight and I would be walking slowly and stiffly. I thought it was because I had been working in an awkward position in a very cold area. Then I started to notice a tremor in my toe and I thought it might be because I had a pinched nerve in my back, so I went to a chiropractor. I was lying on the table in his office with a heat pack on my back when he returned with a book and told me he thought I had Parkinson's.

By August, two different doctors confirmed the chiropractor's hunch. I kept it quiet at first—only my family knew. I didn't know much about Parkinson's, other than what I had noticed by observing the occasional person who had it. Soon after I was told that I had Parkinson's, I decided to change jobs, so I went back to school to become a Nurse Aide. I needed a job that I could do in my later years and I liked working with older people so I figured that it would be a good occupation. I am currently a Home Health Aide, working five days a week, going out to homes to help patients with bathing, feeding and other needs that they may have.

I am on medications, and I exercise and stretch several times a day—sometimes even at patients' houses. My back is my toughest challenge. The pain is best described as what it would feel like if you had a fireplace poker sticking in your back, although stretching is a tremendous help. With God's grace and a back brace I keep working. One other significant symptom for me is that my feet cramp and my toes turn under my foot—when this happens, I cannot even straighten them with my fingers. It is now also hard for me to turn over in bed. If I start walking around before I have taken my medicine, my body is in so much pain that it instantly puts me down on the floor.

I go into homes and I see some people who are just so bitter. One gentleman who had Parkinson's used to run ten miles a day but it seemed he had given up doing anything since his diagnosis. I told him I had Parkinson's, too. He said, "That is too bad—you have my sympathy." I replied, "I don't look at it that way. I feel that Parkinson's has come across my path for a reason. I need to do what I can to help others." He smiled at me after I said that. I noticed that after our conversation, he always seemed to look forward to my visit.

Once a week, I get together with a group of about twenty singers to sing a cappella. The singing has really helped my voice. We are called 'Sisters in Song' and we are affiliated with other choruses that are part of the Sweet Adelines International. Everyone in the choir is just like a sister to me. We have an instructor who keeps us musically in line. Recently, we performed in front of a group of 239 'purple hat' ladies. I also sing with a group called the Monica Stevens Singers *(named after the local founder of the group)*. It is a collection of retired senior citizens—the other singers are mainly in their 70s and early 80s. We go to nursing homes each month to perform a variety of songs and also to try and bring some laughter to the patients.

Jim bought a karaoke machine this summer, and we have started to go to the nursing homes with it. Jim sets up the machine, and I have typed up a list of sing-along sheets that I hand out to the patients. We all sing the older songs together and then I sing some newer songs to them. I was asked what the name of my 'group' was and I answered, "Me, myself and my husband."

I have been writing music since January 2003, and I have recorded a CD called *He Gives My Heart Its Song*. I am self-taught in music writing—I write the lyrics first and I then try to apply the music to what I have written. I also love to write poetry. I was on the Internet in the summer of 2005 and I noticed that there was a creativity contest offered by the World Parkinson Congress. I submitted a poem that was originally written about a patient that I had with Parkinson's who had passed away. I needed a 'little lady' for a picture to represent the initial patient, so I got a good friend of mine, Kate Bradshaw, who was 88 years old, to pose for the picture. I overlaid the poem on a picture of her and then I entered it in the contest. The poem was chosen as one of two winners from Ohio. It was neat, and I was truly tickled when they recognized my little story.

I wanted to attend the 2006 World Parkinson Congress in Washington to learn more about Parkinson's. My husband and I couldn't afford to go far so we borrowed from our trust account in order to get there. I saw a lot of people at the conference with widely ranging conditions and it made me mindful that some people have a tougher challenge with Parkinson's than I do.

I take antioxidants, vitamin E, fish oils and folic acid. I am always examining different natural substances that might prove helpful. Do your research on Parkinson's and don't just leave it up to your doctor.

Being a Home Health Aide constantly reminds me that others are struggling with adversity, too. It gives me perspective. My philosophy is that life is short—so enjoy it! I have a strong faith that has increased since being diagnosed. I firmly believe that God gives me energy and strength. It is up to me to keep a good outlook on life. If I am having a bad day, I remind myself that things will always get better by the next morning. A positive attitude keeps me going.

It is very important to keep moving and I am a firm believer in exercising and stretching. Some mornings I get up and say to myself, "I am so stiff that I don't know if I can make it." But I get down on the floor and stretch with Lilly, my little dog who is a schnauzer/terrier mix. When my feet are finally moving OK, Lilly will often put her paws up in the air and we'll dance around for a bit. By the end of a good stretch and sometimes a dance with Lilly, I am feeling better and ready to go to work.

I can still contribute to making other people's lives happier. I try to encourage people and tell them that things will get better for them. Sometimes I sing to them, which helps to take their mind off their hurt. Help others along life's journey and you will bring a song into someone's life. There is always someone out there that you can assist by lifting their spirits up. Focus on helping them—it will benefit you, too!

I am not going to alter my life and stop doing things that I like to do just because I have Parkinson's.

Patricia Sherrick has not let Parkinson's disease prevent her from doing what she loves. Since being diagnosed, Patricia Sherrick has recorded a CD, and written poetry and stories.

CHAPTER TWENTY-THREE

IAN PEARSON

"I was pulled along through the brush with my legs churning like an eggbeater trying to keep up to him."

Ian Pearson was diagnosed with Parkinson's disease in 1989. He is 56 years old.

On any given flight, there are literally 100 things that can go wrong, such as delays at customs and immigration, issues with baggage, weather factors or problems with connecting flights. It is amazing that planes even get off the ground.

I worked for a total of 22 years at Air Canada, 15 of which were before I was diagnosed with Parkinson's. My wife and I met in 1974 while working there. She walked into our office and I instantly knew that I wanted to marry her. We dated for a couple of years and, in July 1976, we got married and later had a son and a daughter.

In June 1978, a plane to Winnipeg skidded off the runway and went into a ravine and separated in two just by the wing.

I was one of three people who was given the task of phoning all the relatives of the passengers to tell them the status of their loved ones. Although no one died, many of the 105 passengers had crippling injuries. It was one of the most difficult days I ever had at work.

Just before I started to get Parkinson's symptoms, I was made the manager of the reservations office in Toronto. I was responsible for the Air Canada Call Centre and overseeing 350 people. The call centre was as wide as a city block with desks three feet apart. Our number one priority was to make reservations, but we also dealt with complaints or called people to let them know about delayed flights.

In 1987, my right arm started going out straight, almost as if I were walking an imaginary dog. Then my right leg started to drag, and my gait changed. I went to a doctor and he told me it was just stress, so I tried hypnosis and relaxation therapy. I saw some other doctors and was told either that it was all in my head or, as one doctor put it, "I should smarten up."

The period before I was accurately diagnosed was the toughest and very depressing. In 1989, I went back to the first doctor I had consulted. He looked at me as I walked in the door and told me that I did not have to go to the examination room. He said, "You have Parkinson's disease." Finding out I had Parkinson's was an absolute release. I was thinking the worst, like Multiple Sclerosis or a brain tumor, so it was not as worrisome to know I had Parkinson's. I was glad to be able to go back and tell my staff what I had because they had been worried about my condition.

Early on I was given Sinemet which worked very well for me. Taking Sinemet and having a clear conscience because

I was not keeping my health a secret led to me having some very productive years at work. I was told that I would have a honeymoon period with the Sinemet and that it would be good for five to eight years. They were right. After seven years, I started to gyrate a bit. Sometimes I would freeze when someone would hold a door for me and I would not be able to get through the door. That was really embarrassing. I would try and explain it but people would just look at me strangely.

Close to the end of my tenure at Air Canada, I was phoned on a Friday afternoon by a Vice President. He told that they were going to have a massive reduction in management staff and that I would have to fire 12 of my 15 supervisors on Monday. I was told that my job would be to get them from the main floor up to the personnel department. They would process them from there and then call me when the next person was to come up. On that Monday, I took the most senior supervisor up and, by about half way through the day, the place was just numb. Agents were not taking calls, people were in tears, and my Parkinson's symptoms—which were exacerbated by stress—were on full display. I felt like a duck that day—I was calm on the top of the water but down below I was paddling like heck. I started to feel that I could no longer cope with the high stress of my job. I was afraid they were going to fire me. I retired in 1996 because my productivity had been going down and I had challenges with multitasking.

In 1999, my neurologist tipped me off to a program called Independent Dogs Incorporated *(IDI)*, which was a program put on by SmithKline Beecham that provided trained service dogs to help people with mobility challenges. They had ten dogs in the United States and they had decided to add one more for someone in Canada. I said I was interested. I was a good candidate because of my age and the fact that I had a strong voice. I was falling more, so I thought that a dog would be a good help.

I was given a dog named Pax, which is Latin for Peace. He is a black Labrador retriever and a very large dog. Pax has helped me to overcome a social stigma when out in public. Previously, if I was alone and stumbling about because my walking was not very good, people would give me a wide berth. I hated the fact that they were thinking, "This guy is crazy or drunk—stay away from him." Now, when I have Pax with me I do not get those same looks.

I have a big harness on Pax, so if I stumble I can usually keep my feet. If I fall, I just have to yell the command, "Brace!" When he hears that command, Pax will come by and stand sideways—I then can put my hand on his back and get up.

When Pax's harness is on he is a service dog. When it comes off, he reverts back to being a regular dog. One time when Pax and I were in training, I did everything wrong—I attached his leash but did not put the harness on him. I took him for a walk and did not realize he saw a squirrel. Suddenly, he took off after the squirrel. I had only the leash to control him, so I was pulled along through the brush with my legs churning like an eggbeater trying to keep up to him. Imagine a six-foot dog standing on his back legs excitedly looking up a tree. The squirrel kept on climbing to the top of the tree, so Pax finally just gave up. I took Pax from the tree and finally had him sitting down, but in less than ten minutes he was off again chasing a robin around.

I don't take anything for granted. I am more compassionate now and I am very sympathetic to others, especially those with young-onset Parkinson's and older individuals with more advanced cases. I feel Parkinson's patients have a higher level of empathy and that our sympathetic nervous system is more finely tuned but also more fragile.

I believe there are a lot of people that are not coming out with the fact they have Parkinson's or who are keeping a low profile. I live in Mississauga, a city with a population in excess of 600,000. By my calculations, there should be at least 2,000 people with Parkinson's in the city. One would never guess that the number is that high simply because one doesn't see many individuals with Parkinson's out in public.

Don't let anything go so far that it becomes a real problem to overcome—especially depression. I had depression badly just before I was diagnosed back in 1989. It was like being in a deep, dark tunnel where my head felt like a rock in the middle of the tunnel. Depression makes you feel weak and that is not the case at all. It is not a weakness—it is an illness. If you start to feel depressed, you need to seek treatment immediately. If you don't, then you could get into a whole lot of trouble that could be much worse than Parkinson's.

There is a purpose to everything that happens to us. The choices we make determine where we end up. I believe we are here for a reason. We are on a journey—some journeys are long and arduous while others may be short-lived, but we all have a purpose.

The chance to live our lives is a gift we all have.

Ian Pearson is involved with the Mississauga Parkinson's chapter and Parkinson's advocacy. His goal for the

chapter is to raise one million dollars over ten years—
$100,000 per year. This year they raised $89,000.

Ian Pearson was one of the first people in North America
to have a dog to assist him with his balance. He wrote a
book in 1999 called Crossroads, *which details his*
experience training his service dog Pax.

CHAPTER TWENTY-FOUR

MAGDA SCHIJFF

"I could finally beat my husband to the newspaper."

Magda Schijff was diagnosed with Parkinson's disease in 2001. She is 54 years old.

Ever since I was a little girl I loved nursing. I would go with my mother to pick up my older sisters after their nursing shifts. In the car I used to snuggle into them and smell the antiseptic from the hospital. They would bring me syringes from the hospital, which I used to inject water into every one of my mother's plants. I went on to Chapel Hill, North Carolina and worked as a nurse at Duke from 1974 until 1977, at which point I took a two-year leave of absence to earn my Bachelor of Science in Nursing degree.

I paid my way through school and I was very poor as a result. My father gave me money in a roundabout way—he had people who owed money to his business over the years so he challenged me to collect the overdue funds. I was allowed to keep anything that I recovered—I became pretty good at collecting the money!

All I could afford was an attic apartment. My food budget was $7 per week and my diet consisted of apples, eggs, cookies and cream for my coffee. As a result, I often visited friends at mealtime! After graduating, I moved to a larger, two-storey house in the middle of a trailer park. If someone had lit a match to it, the house would have been gone in two seconds flat. My landlord used to leave moonshine at the door—we had great parties there.

In 1985, I got married at the age of 32. We had kids soon after. It was a hectic time—I remember working a twelve-hour shift, making dinner, and buying groceries just before having my third child. With the addition of the third we were outnumbered and totally swamped. Raising three boys born in three and a half years was a major feat. They loved sports, especially lacrosse, rugby and soccer. We had 'movie night' every Friday evening complete with popcorn. My children were the main focus in my life.

My symptoms started to appear in 1991. I began to hold my left arm close to my body and, when I walked, my arm was crooked and not swinging freely. I could not figure out why. People started to notice that I was limping slightly. I also began to have lower back pain. Then I realized that I could not pick up my left foot at times and also that my left hand was unable to type on a computer keyboard.

I started seeing many different doctors late in 1994, after experiencing three years of symptoms. The doctors did an X-ray and MRI of my neck and said that I had cervical spinal stenosis. I had two surgeries to solve the problem—the first one did not work out, but two years later I had a second operation and it was more effective. I was out of work for a year between the surgeries and in terrible pain. In retrospect, I may or may not have needed the operations.

After ten years of symptoms, I was diagnosed with Parkinson's disease in 2001. My husband was relieved to know what it was because he believed that you can deal with anything as long as you know what you have to deal with—I was not relieved. I was down and I had to take antidepressants. I was really, really stubborn and wouldn't admit to what was happening. I tried to internalize it. For a while, I made it horrible for my husband and my family to be around me. Eventually, I realized I could not hide my Parkinson's. I felt better once I let people know what was happening with me.

One side effect of the medications that I took led to a serious problem. I was into knitting and ended up continually buying yarn—enough to literally fill a room in a house. I got mesmerized by the different colors and textures. After years of looking after kids, I rationalized that I needed to pamper myself. I was devious and took $20 here and $20 there, trying to hide my spending. All the while, I was depleting the family savings. I couldn't stop the addictive desire to spend. Fortunately, I changed one med for another and that took away the spending urges a bit. I still love knitting, but I am not quite as obsessed with it.

Duke was very good to me in that they found jobs that I could do with my limitations. I was a nurse coordinator and helped to oversee a multimillion dollar renovation. When that was completed in 2002, I went on disability.

My left foot has been broken four times since 2001. I never realized the dystonia of Parkinson's was causing me to step on my toes instead of my heels. I finally had botox injected into my foot in 2003 to help relax the spasms and relieve the dystonia. My foot doesn't work any better—but at least it's younger looking!

I had been approached about deep brain stimulation *(DBS)* surgery, but I thought that I did not need anyone mucking with my brain. My symptoms finally progressed to a point where I had difficulty walking, muscle pain, and dyskinesia. I was becoming so focused on myself that I was losing time with my family. I decided I should try the operation and so I had DBS surgery in July 2006. In retrospect, it was the best thing I could have done.

The operation took just under five hours. They cut off my hair on one side and I could feel the drill putting holes into my head. Surprisingly, that did not seem to bother me that much—it was just a weird sensation. They had me wear a 'hot-wired' glove on my left hand and asked me to perform tasks including playing video games so that they could pinpoint the exact area of the brain to place the wires. I was in the hospital overnight and home the next day. After the operation, it was exhilarating and thrilling. Once again, I had energy and was expressive. I could finally beat my husband to the newspaper.

You need to see the humor in life. The first time I actually laughed about Parkinson's was on a Christmas morning a few years ago when I opened a small package lovingly bought for me by my husband. It was a flashlight that did not require batteries. My husband enthusiastically explained to me that all I had to do was shake it repeatedly to power it up. A vision flashed through my head of a dark world being lit up and saved by a large diverse group of shaky people with Parkinson's who were aiming and shaking the lights while croaking out the song *We Are The World.*

Don't isolate yourself. My girlfriends have been a terrific support network for me. We have been friends since the 70s and experienced a lot together. Find a good medical team that you can relate to and keep a log of your Parkinson's meds, symptoms, and treatments. I am pigheaded and I believe one should never give in to Parkinson's.

If I die tomorrow, I am comfortable that I have experienced all that I have wanted in life. I have loved, I have laughed, and I have lost. I feel like I have had a very full life. Except for the excessive spending on yarn, I have no regrets. I want to see my children fully grown and married and I want to grow old with my husband, but I am also preparing for things in case I don't.

I have a wonderful family and I am feeling closer to them than I ever have. My relationship with my husband took a dive after the Parkinson's diagnosis, during the period when I was in denial, but it has since improved and it is now very solid. He has been very strong, and I now try to consciously do more for him. Don't forget your spouse or primary caregiver and be there for him or her just as they have been there for you.

Support is not one-sided.

Magda Schijff is feeling much better as a result of her DBS surgery. She stays busy looking after her family, exercising and helping out in the community.

CHAPTER TWENTY-FIVE

JOHN SURRATT

"Parkinson's makes people become more resourceful."

John Surratt was diagnosed with Parkinson's disease in 1996. He is 95 years old.

My first job was working in the late 1920s with film people in a business that was across the road from my high school in Dallas. I think I was getting paid about 25 cents an hour. It was a freelance operation whose principal business was to film news which would be shown during the time between the features in the theaters. I was very interested in editing the sounds on film. Everything had to be done exactly right and if you messed up, the people on the screen talked after their lips moved.

My wife lived a block away from where I grew up and we knew each other through grade school and high school. We got married in 1932 and we had two little girls, nine years apart. I left the film business after the Great Depression and

I became a grease monkey for the Magnolia Petroleum Company, who had some high-end, fancy filling stations.

I was very much interested in radio communications and its capabilities. At the time, the police department only had one-way radios and if their cars didn't run continuously the batteries ran down. While working in the filling station, I discovered a way to solve that problem. I made a radio that would pick up the signals without the car having to run, which attracted a lot of police. It became common practice for the police to drive up to our filling station driveway and then turn off their cars and use my radio. I ended up applying for an opening in the police department and became a policeman for a time.

After the Second World War, I moved into the aviation industry. I could not resist aviation as I had been building scale planes and models as a hobby. I became a civilian aviator for the military, testing techniques on how to better teach humans to use airplanes. I eventually worked at a location near Greenville, Texas on a secret espionage project converting the insides of aircrafts like the B-29, C-130 and other later model transports into flying rooms full of highly sophisticated electronic equipment. We thought the project was a big secret, yet the tails of the airplanes were so large you could see them from the highway. One of us got a little bit smart and put some canvas over the tails to hide them but by then word was out.

My job was to show the GIs how to use the equipment. The goal was to be able to have the modified planes measure how fast the Russians could scramble their planes after we flew over their border, hopefully before they would shoot us down. One of the dozen or so aircraft we modified was shot down in Russian territory—this was kept secret.

After retiring in 1969, I wanted to be able to track the satellites I had been involved with earlier in my life, so I bought a twenty-foot satellite dish and had it put in my backyard. My intent was to pick up radio signals—which wasn't what the dish was originally designed to do, but with a few little modifications it worked just fine and had tracking capabilities. It outdid what I expected even though some things backfired. It was a big sensation for a long time but finally the neighbors accepted it as part of the landscape. I ended up helping the Dallas Police Department by working as a radio operator at my home using my dish.

One time, I was walking down the street with a piece of paper in my left hand and the paper was shaking. I didn't think the wind was strong enough to do that and I soon realized that it was my hand that was causing the shaking. That symptom really got my attention—and it led me to see my family doctor who in turn sent me to a specialist. In 1996, I was told that I had Parkinson's. The specialist who diagnosed me said, "In five years I will give you some medicine, but until then just keep going like you are."

When I found out that I had Parkinson's disease, I was worried to no end. I had a friend named Joe Bibby who was a famous Second World War pilot who also had Parkinson's. I spent my whole day pumping him with questions and he answered every one of them. He said, "All the medicine in the world won't do near as much good as physical therapy will." His advice has worked for me!

I have one patent for inventing an airway door with stairs on it. It was picked up by an airline and, although I didn't make any major funds from it, I did make enough to justify my fooling around with it. I have always been inventing, and I am currently working on three or four inventions right now.

I am trying to figure out how I can develop a method to detect when a Parkinson's person is going to fall. When the person is about to fall, a device that has an airbag would be inflated, and then they would land on something soft. I don't know how successful I will be, but I am still trying to work at it. Parkinson's makes people more resourceful.

I always try to get people with Parkinson's to go to support groups. One advantage of support groups is that you meet a lot of other people who are going through the same situation. I sympathize with the younger ones who get it because they also have to deal with things like the cost of insurance and job risks. A big load also falls on the caregivers. My goal is to spread the word about Parkinson's. There is a lot more that can be done. There are a lot of prominent people who have it who could help others by stepping forward.

At this point in time I have just about all the symptoms. I am past the stage of walking—I scooter around now. Shaking is a very minor item with me. I have lost my sense of balance and, as of right now, I am up to nine times that I have fallen today. This is why I am working very hard and diligently on this airbag idea.

Help is very much needed by a lot of people. About one and a half years ago, I had a grandson whose wife and his three little boys were out on the curb. He had lost his job and everything, and he was an alcoholic. I took him in. Fifteen months later he was sober and he had gone back to work and moved out from living with me. I think that group of three little boys stimulated me more than anything I have done in the last ten years. I could not keep up with them. They were a lively group! I knew that they needed some help badly and I was glad that I could give them assistance.

The best advice I ever received in my life was to "keep my mouth shut and listen." That is hard to do! I also try to find a humorous side to every tragic event I am involved with. It doesn't always work, but sometimes it works quite well. Every negative thing also has a positive side, too. For instance, if I am serving at the table and you want some potatoes, I don't have to shake the spoon to get the potatoes off—the Parkinson's does it for me.

You can always find something positive to focus on.

John Surratt lived on his own for 95 years and only recently has moved into an assisted living facility. In November 2005, the Dallas Police Department gave John Surratt an award for 3,000 volunteer work hours in his neighborhood.

CHAPTER TWENTY-SIX

ROBBIE TUCKER

"How many times can you visit the doctor and leave with Tylenol?"

Robbie Tucker was diagnosed with Parkinson's disease in June 2005. He is 29 years old.

I was born in 1977 in a small town called White Rapids, New Brunswick. My mom was a Registered Nursing Assistant and after my brother and I were born, she became a full-time, stay-at-home mom. My dad was a truck driver who delivered fuel in New Brunswick and Nova Scotia. He was hard-working and musically talented—he liked to play guitar in his spare time.

When I was 12 years old, I remember visiting my mother at the hospital and seeing this really nice room at the end of the hall. I asked the nurse, "What is this room for and why is it nicer than the rest?" The nurse told me that the room was where they put people who would not go home and who were likely going to die. The next day I came to the hospital and my mother was in that room. She had cancer, and was in tremendous pain and on morphine in her last days, but she never gave up or complained. My mother was the most positive person I have ever met. She would ask us how we were, how school was, did our father make us a good lunch and so on. She died of cancer on September 12, 1989.

After my mother died, I was alone in the house a lot because my older brother had his own friends and my dad was often on the road driving. In that period of my life, I shut myself away from everyone. I didn't listen to music seriously until I purchased my first Elvis tape. I am not sure why I bought it, but I wore it out playing *Blue Suede Shoes* over and over. It was very special to listen to—it was so different from anything else that I heard in the early 90s. I began to spend most of my free time singing in my room. From the moment that I started listening to that Elvis tape, I decided that I wanted to be a musician.

I went to work at a pizza place after graduating from high school in 1995. I was living day to day because I never had any real career plans after high school. Music was my entire focus. I started writing songs in grade nine, although I had never had any formal music lessons other than the rudimentary courses in high school. After Elvis, I was heavily influenced by the operatic voice of Roy Orbison. I got into his music so much that I think I lost friends over it, as they would always hear the same Roy Orbison songs if they were around me.

In between working in the pizza place or at various restaurants, I continued to try to write and record songs using our crappy stereo. By 2003 I had written some songs so, in April of that year, I produced and released my very first album, *The*

Ledden Street Sessions. I taught myself all of the instruments and played them myself on that album. I didn't know what anybody would think of it because no one had ever heard any of my stuff before. The album went OK.

In January 2004, I started working at a restaurant in Halifax called Jungle Jim's. I didn't really want to do it but I needed money and it was part of the same restaurant chain that I had worked at while I was at home, so there was nothing new to learn. We used to have contests there to see who could roll knives and forks into a napkin the fastest. I used to be really fast but now when I tried to do it, my hands would slow down and then finally they would stop moving. At this place we also had to mix our own drinks, and I was so slow—I couldn't figure out why. It got awkward when my arms wouldn't move as well, so I would put my hands in my pockets. I told my friend about what I was experiencing and he thought I was just low on vitamins. I went to the hospital in Halifax a few times and saw three or four different doctors. I had an MRI done but nothing showed up, so they just told me that I needed to rest and relax because there was nothing wrong with me.

That summer, I put a band together and we toured a bit, playing to smallish crowds. When we were touring, we liked to switch instruments to show how versatile the band was and I found out then that I could no longer play any instruments other than the guitar. I didn't care that I was slow when rolling the knives and forks into napkins at Jungle Jim's because I hated the job, but when this mystery illness started to affect something I loved to do, it was a different story. It was the worst time of my life.

I was tested so many times for this and that. I would always leave with no answer, wondering what was wrong with me.

One doctor, after hearing about my mother dying, even said "Maybe it is something psychological." That made me so angry! I said to him, "My mother died 17 years ago and now I can't walk or use my hands—now that makes perfect sense." How many times can you visit the doctor and leave with Tylenol? I just needed to know that I was not going nuts and that something was actually wrong with me.

It got so bad that I couldn't perform live anymore. I remember playing a song for my friends and we videotaped it, but it was too painful to watch. The video showed me taking the guitar out of the case, moving in what seemed like slow motion and having no emotion or power in my voice. However, inside my apartment, whenever I felt good, I could still record. I decided that I would try to make another album and I spent the next eight months recording. The result was an album that was called *Songs from apartment #12*. If I had not had my music to get me through this time, I do not know how well I would have done. I was determined not to let whatever was wrong with me stop me from making music.

Each day I would look up different symptoms on the Internet, and I would always end up reading about Parkinson's. The trouble in researching things was that many of my symptoms were general and applicable to other diseases. I also went to the gym five times per week and forced myself to do an hour of cardio. I would literally have to hold onto things as I was walking home because I was so tired. I was trying everything to fix the mystery problem.

On my third visit to my current neurologist, he and his associate agreed that it looked like I had young-onset Parkinson's. It was in June 2005 that I finally got my first Parkinson's medication. I told my dad and, while initially he was at a loss for words, he has been really helpful and supportive ever since. Ironically, an intern who had examined me one year earlier had asked me if anyone in my family had Parkinson's. No one in my family has had it but the weird thing is that in the tiny area where I grew up, three or four people have it now.

The meds are working really well. My voice feels much stronger and it sounds a lot better. I have a good outlook, but if I didn't have the medication I would not be as positive. I am grateful to have the chance to live again. Before Parkinson's, I would get up in the morning and shower. The only difference is that now I have to also take pills. It is not a big deal.

If your meds are working OK then you have an opportunity to live your life for the next ten minutes or for the next five years. I think it is important to find something in life that gives you a reason to live. For me, that is music and art. Find out what that 'something' is and then focus your energy on it. Don't dwell on your problems, otherwise all your energy will be centered on the wrong thing. If you have something in life you like to do, then do it now.

I don't know how long I am here for, and I don't want to know. However, as long as I am here I am going to make music and nothing is going to stop me. Sometimes, something might get in my way—but nothing will ever stop me.

I have to have a positive outlook on life because there is no reason why I shouldn't.

Robbie Tucker has now recorded 35 songs—including a duet with his father. He also wrote a song called **PD**

Groove, *which is his jab at Parkinson's disease.*

Robbie Tucker continues to record and his newest song, The Carnival *was the 2006 Canadian runner-up for Music Aid, The International Music Awards.*

CHAPTER TWENTY-SEVEN

JANET RENO

"I resolved never to 'just stand by'."

Janet Reno was diagnosed with Parkinson's disease in October 1995. She is 68 years old.

I never dreamed that I would one day have the opportunity to become the Attorney General for the United States. It was an incredible experience to find myself walking into the basement of the White House without identification and going up to the second floor for meetings. It was something that I never got over. It didn't seem possible—but it was. I found the whole experience of being the Attorney General rewarding.

In the Department of Justice, you learn that making progress in crime prevention takes time. I believe that starting crime prevention early on in people's lives makes a difference because then you can have them begin on the right foot. Immigration is a difficult area because there are so many conflicts—but I think it is imperative that this nation never forget that it is a nation of immigrants and that is where our strength comes from.

Being criticized—both fairly and unfairly—comes with the job of being the Attorney General. My father was a newspaper reporter and my mother was a freelance reporter. They taught me that people are going to say bad things about you and if you are going to let it bother you then you should get a different job.

My first symptoms appeared in March of 1995. I had an apartment two blocks from The Mall, near the Department of Justice. I walked around that area each morning at about 6 o'clock, for a half-hour or so. One day as I was walking, I found that my thumb and forefinger came together in an odd way—it was definitely unusual. I started inquiring about what it could be. It looked like it might be Parkinson's so, in October of 1995, I visited a neurologist, who diagnosed me with it. I knew of Parkinson's and I understood that there was shaking associated with it but, beyond that, I did not know much about the disease at all.

I was determined to have full public disclosure of the fact that I had been diagnosed with Parkinson's. My doctors also made themselves publicly available to answer questions about the disease and how it would affect me. I wanted people, including President Clinton, to tell me if they thought it would impair my ability to do the job in any way—no one ever indicated that it would. Everyone was very supportive.

When I walked across Pennsylvania Avenue for the last time as Attorney General, on January 20, 2001, President Bush was being sworn in. I felt a great weight being lifted off my shoulders—then a dark cloud appeared. I realized I had one more thing to do. I thought to myself, "You haven't <u>really</u> agreed to be on Saturday Night Live tonight, have you?"

Two hours later, I walked into NBC and there was Will Ferrell, wearing my blue suit *(Will Ferrell occasionally parodied Janet Reno on Saturday Night Live. On January 20, 2001, Janet Reno appeared as herself in the skit, 'Janet Reno's Dance Party')*. Will Ferrell's mother, aunt, in-laws and wife were there, too. It was a large collection of individuals reveling in humor. I am so glad my colleagues and my nieces and nephews persuaded me to be on the show—it was great fun!

In 2002, I ran for Governor of Florida. I was very disturbed at the status and the lack of action with respect to issues that related to abused and neglected children, the school system, the health care system, and our environment. When I was campaigning, people were saying that I would not be able to do the job because of the Parkinson's. One lady, a 90-year-old retired educator, said "I know her hand shakes, but I don't care about her hand. I care about her head—and her head is just fine, thank you." I knew that running for Governor was going to be a difficult campaign, but I am glad I got involved and ran because it gave me a chance to try and change things, and also to challenge people to resolve these problems.

Back in the early 1950s, I had an opportunity to spend a year in Germany with my uncle, who had been an Allied High Commission judge during the occupation. One day he took me past the Dachau concentration camp before it had been opened to the public, and he told me what had happened there. That night, I asked the German people with whom I was staying and whose friendship I had acquired,

"How could you let this happen?" And they replied, "We just stood by—we just stood by."

Ever since then, I resolved never to 'just stand by'. I am very interested in the Innocence Project and post-conviction DNA testing that has resulted in the exoneration of people who have been convicted of serious crimes and who have served substantial jail terms or faced the death penalty. I want to do all I can do to contribute to efforts that make sure that innocent people do not get charged and, if they do get charged, that they are found not guilty.

My brother has also been diagnosed with Parkinson's. We drank well water while growing up, and I think that this common factor might have played a role in the development of Parkinson's for both my brother and me.

I keep asking people why we don't organize information registries for Parkinson's. There is a lot of data out there that has not been collected, and we could learn so much if we kept statistics on the many different aspects of Parkinson's disease. Some individuals say that there is not enough scientific certainty on factors that could contribute to Parkinson's, but I think that they should at least let the people know the statistics on things like well water, pesticides, or working in a certain industry. I think we should let people make judgments for themselves based on all the information available.

The tremor in my left hand has now become more pronounced, and my right hand has been affected, too—my handwriting is lousy. I also tire more easily. One of my challenges is that I have arthritis. If I did not have it, the Parkinson's would be a lot easier to deal with. The arthritis which affects me the most in the knees is currently bothering me more than the Parkinson's—but that changes week to week.

Despite the arthritis, I have learned how to step in and out of a kayak. Last spring, I kayaked on the Potomac as well as the Shenandoah and James Rivers. It is a very good workout.

Parkinson's treats everyone it hits differently and what applies to me might not apply to you. There are a lot of people out there with Parkinson's who get up every day and go to work and do their job. They are making a difference, and they will be able to do that for five or ten more years. There are many positive things to be doing.

Life is an interconnected journey. I think that each experience provides its own challenges that you can learn from. One of the hardest things to do is to develop and maintain a sense of hope—yet, at the same time to be realistic that there are impacts of this disease that are devilishly difficult to cope with. However, the more someone tries, the more they will succeed in overcoming the disease. Don't be disappointed. If you fail at something, pick yourself up and try again.

A sense of hope, held in a realistic way, is something that all Parkinson's patients can develop and share.

Janet Reno was the 78th Attorney General of the United States, serving from 1993 through 2001. She was the first woman to have the title of Attorney General, and also the longest serving Attorney General in the history of the United States. Under her leadership, the Department of Justice managed high profile cases involving the Oklahoma City bombing, the World Trade Center bombing, antitrust actions against Microsoft, the

Branch Davidians, the Montana Freemen, Elio Gonzalez and the Unabomber.

Janet Reno delivers speeches a few times each month. She is actively working with the Innocence Project (a non-profit legal clinic that—as of February 2007—had freed 194 individuals who were wrongfully convicted) and she is also helping to raise awareness for Parkinson's disease.

CHAPTER TWENTY-EIGHT

BILL BARNEWITZ

"Parkinson's was a wake-up call telling me to make the absolute most out of my time."

Bill Barnewitz was diagnosed with Parkinson's disease in 2001. He is 48 years old.

Music was a central feature of our daily life in Reno. My mother is an accomplished pianist and my father was a musician early in his life. At one point I sang in a boys choir and I was convinced that I was going to be an opera singer. Of course, it takes real ability to do that and, as it turns out, I had no real talent for singing. I could carry a tune, but after my voice changed, I didn't have a beautiful voice in any shape or form.

I heard a visiting orchestra come to Reno and I was just stunned by how beautiful the French horn sounded. Right from that point, I knew that was what I wanted to do. It was a moment when I had tunnel vision—all I saw was the row of horns playing. It was like a light bulb being turned on.

Since then, the French horn has always been my only focus for an instrument.

I went to the North Carolina School of the Arts and then I attended The Julliard School of Music before playing in New York City for a while. Then I got a job in California in an orchestra that turned out to be failing financially, so I started to look for something else to do. I went to work in a winery and quit playing the horn for two years.

Another light bulb went on when I was working at the winery and sitting inside a ten thousand gallon stainless steel tank, cleaning tannic acid off the sides of the tank with a combination of citric acid and cold water. I was listening to a radio that was playing New World Symphony and I thought to myself, "Listen to those horns—I can play better than that." I got my horn out again, and I found that the Utah Symphony had an opening so I auditioned for it. I was with the Utah Symphony for ten years and that's also where I met my wife.

In 1995, the Milwaukee Symphony was auditioning for a principal horn. They had three large auditions and could not find anybody. Then they started inviting people and they called me. I hadn't thought two seconds about moving to Milwaukee prior to that. In September I played with the orchestra for a week and auditioned for the committee, but then I forgot about it, because the auditioning process was very spread out. I was offered the job in December. We moved to Milwaukee with our twin girls and it ended up being a very good choice.

Much of the music we play is so much fun to share with the audience. Each week, there are at least two or three concerts and three or four rehearsals. Besides playing horn in the orchestra, I also teach about nine hours a week at Northwestern University and a few hours at home. I almost never stop practicing. In my head, I'm always going over music, mentally thinking about how I want to phrase things or how I want to practice stuff the next time I pick up the horn. In some ways, music is a very selfish and all-encompassing business because it takes so much time to practice and perform.

My symptoms first started to show about six years ago. They began with cramping in my left foot. Then a small tremor appeared in my left leg that would not have been noticeable to anyone else. My wife was more concerned initially—she has an uncanny sense about her and she thought I might have Parkinson's. I went through the usual route of things with my regular family physician, just asking what she thought. She ordered a battery of tests and none of those showed anything. The doctor that conducted all the nerve tests recommended that I should go see Dr. Nausieda at the Parkinson's Center here in Milwaukee, and for him it seemed like an easy diagnosis. I didn't really know anything about Parkinson's at the time. I mean, I knew it existed, but only that.

At first, there was a psychological aspect to how Parkinson's would affect my playing. Learning how to time my medications and get the dosages just right was a big challenge for a year. I think I was incorrectly predicting a shorter lifespan of being able to play after this diagnosis. I mean, I felt a little bit like Chicken Little—"The sky is falling!" It was easy at the beginning to assume the worst. But it was also easy to change my thinking and tell myself, "You've given music up before, but now you're back in it for the right reasons and the right reasons are because you love the music. So just keep that in mind and take care of yourself. Love the music and just keep going for as long as you can."

My family life gives me the most joy of anything that I do. Our girls and my wife are all animal nuts. We have two dogs, a cat, a hedgehog and a frog, so I get 'pet therapy' as well. My family's support has been huge. There was also great communal support from the orchestra when I told them I had Parkinson's. Being in an orchestra is like having an additional 88 people in your family.

I think you should contact your doctors when you notice a change, and I think you should keep in touch with them on some kind of regular basis. But in between visits, you should learn as much about Parkinson's as possible, so that if you are noticing something different, you can mark it and report it. I'm not exactly the poster child for exercise but I know that it's important. I also feel that it is essential to have someone to talk to when you're not feeling good about how things are going because I think it's easy to get the element of depression involved. You don't always need to talk to a therapist or anyone professional—it is just as easy to say to a friend, "I'm not happy about how things are going and do you want to go for a walk?"

These days, I have a lot more tremors and fatigue. But the medication really works. I take my Sinemet and I go about my day. As long as it's effective, I'm satisfied to keep going the same way.

The idea of eventually changing careers does not bother me in the least because I've done it before and I know it's entirely possible. Music is a wonderful thing, but there will still be concerts to attend and recordings to listen to, so it's not like I would be without music. There are so many other interesting things to do and, if I'm not too disabled, I'm going to have a great time doing them. If I am too disabled, then I'm still going to find something to do with my brain to keep it busy. I've thought about this a lot because there will be a point at which I can't play anymore.

I do not want to be known as 'The horn player with Parkinson's'. I want to be known as a good horn player—with no conditions attached. I don't want to let Parkinson's define me. I think that is important and it probably applies to any disease that someone may be fighting. Don't let the disease define you.

I have a student whose father has very severe Multiple Sclerosis *(MS)*, and when I think of his life being actually physically cut short by MS, it reminds me that there are a lot worse things than having Parkinson's. Which is not to say that Parkinson's is great because it isn't at all. But you can live with Parkinson's. You can keep going for a long time—you can do the same things you were doing before. You just notice that you're not feeling as tiptop as you were before you had symptoms.

If you want your life to be all that it can be, then don't dwell on the fact that you have Parkinson's but instead dwell on the fact that, until you are really disabled, you should make the most out of your life. Parkinson's was a wake-up call telling me to make the absolute most out of my time. That's the thing, isn't it? No matter who you are or what you're diagnosed with, or even if you are never diagnosed with anything, you should treasure life and be fully engaged in it.

Bill Barnewitz is the principal horn player with the Milwaukee Symphony and the Santa Fe Opera orchestra. He is currently working on a horn and chamber music CD that will include other instruments and singers, too. All the proceeds are going to go to Parkinson's research and education. Bill Barnewitz hopes to have the CD ready for the public by May 2007.

APPENDIX
ADDITIONAL SOURCES OF INFORMATION

For further information on any of the individuals who have been profiled in *Surviving Adversity–living with Parkinson's disease*, please see below.

Chapter One:
Davis Phinney
Davis Phinney Foundation
www.davisphinneyfoundation.com

Chapter Two:
Pat Hull
www.SurvivingAdversity.com

Chapter Three:
Books:
Knowlton Nash
The Microphone Wars
Kennedy and Diefenbaker
Cue the Elephant!
Trivia Pursuit
Swashbucklers
History on the Run
Visions of Canada
Prime Time at Ten
Times to Remember
www.SurvivingAdversity.com

Chapter Four:
Book:
John Ball
Living Well, Running Hard
www.teamparkinsonla.org

Chapter Five:
Books:
Janet Sinke
Ten Lessons Learned
Grandma's Treasure Chest
I Wanna Go to Grandma's House
Grandpa's Fishin' Friend
Grandma's Christmas Tree
www.mygrandmaandme.com

Chapter Six:	**Raul Yzaguirre** www.SurvivingAdversity.com
Chapter Seven:	**Louise Whitney** www.SurvivingAdversity.com
Chapter Eight:	**Bill Commans** www.SurvivingAdversity.com
Chapter Nine:	**Chris Olsen** www.SurvivingAdversity.com
Chapter Ten:	**Irv Popkin** www.SurvivingAdversity.com
Chapter Eleven:	**Margaret Hansell** www.SurvivingAdversity.com
Chapter Twelve:	**Steve Bohannon** Selected Poems www.pdyoungatheartsupportgroup.org
Chapter Thirteen:	**Shelby Hayter** Pass The Baton for Parkinson's www.ohri.ca/prc/
Chapter Fourteen:	**John Thomas** www.SurvivingAdversity.com
Chapter Fifteen:	**Linda Cooper** www.SurvivingAdversity.com
Chapter Sixteen: **Book:**	**Dr. David Heydrick** The Parkinson's Pyramid – *coming Sept 2007* www.SurvivingAdversity.com
Chapter Seventeen:	**Patty Meehan** www.SurvivingAdversity.com
Chapter Eighteen:	**Nick Kaethler** www.SurvivingAdversity.com

Chapter Nineteen:	**Tom O'Donnell** www.SurvivingAdversity.com
Chapter Twenty:	**Cherie Zaun** www.SurvivingAdversity.com
Chapter Twenty-One:	**Carroll Neesemann** www.SurvivingAdversity.com
Chapter Twenty-Two: CD:	**Patricia Sherrick** He Gives My Heart Its Song
Poetry:	The Little Lady and the Lord www.SurvivingAdversity.com
Chapter Twenty-Three:	**Ian Pearson** www.SurvivingAdversity.com
Chapter Twenty-Four:	**Magda Schijff** www.SurvivingAdversity.com
Chapter Twenty-Five:	**John Surratt** www.SurvivingAdversity.com
Chapter Twenty-Six: CDs:	**Robbie Tucker** **The Ledden Street Sessions** **Songs from apartment #12** www.robbietucker.com
Chapter Twenty-Seven:	**Janet Reno** www.SurvivingAdversity.com
Chapter Twenty-Eight: CD:	**Bill Barnewitz** **Long Road Home** www.wiparkinson.org

To order

SURVIVING ADVERSITY—
living with Parkinson's
disease

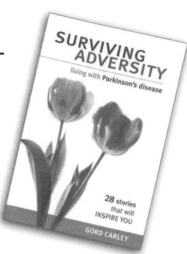

OR

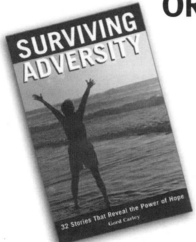

SURVIVING ADVERSITY—
The Collection

Single copy price
US $15 / CAN $17 + shipping and handling

Custom Printed Copies—Surviving Adversity can be
customized for fundraising purposes. Please call for more
details.

Order online at www.SurvivingAdversity.com
or call 1-866-220-4909